A Nurse's Guide to Public Speaking

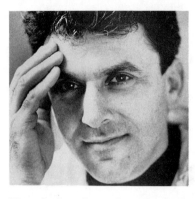**Barry Jay Kaplan** is a free-lance health and medical writer who has been published in many trade and consumer publications, including *Physicians' Money Digest, Oncology Times, Medica, Emergency Medicine, The New Physician, Physicians' Travel, Health and Science, Physician,* and *Your Healthy Best.* He worked as a writer in the Division of Nursing at Columbia Presbyterian Hospital, where he observed organization of community medical and social work offices and co-wrote *The Influence Factor,* with the Executive Vice President of Nursing, Kathleen Dirschl, PhD, on the role she played in the decentralized organization. He also compiled and edited the *Nurses' Educational Guide* as part of the Penzance Foundation grant. He worked at Brookdale University Hospital Medical Center as a writer in the Community Affairs office, where he wrote several annual reports and the Residency brochures for Medical School. He has written extensively on the subject of depression and produced a series of newsletters for Pfizer. He has also written for Montefiore Hospital, New York Hospital, St. Lukes-Roosevelt Hospital, and SUNY Health Science Center in Brooklyn. In addition to his work in the health and medical fields, Mr. Kaplan is a playwright whose plays have been produced in theaters across the country and in London. He is also the author of the best-selling novels *Black Orchid* (with Nicholas Meyer) and *Biscayne.* He has a Master of Fine Arts degree in writing from the University of Iowa Writers' Workshop.

A Nurse's Guide to Public Speaking

BARRY JAY KAPLAN, MFA

 Springer Publishing Company

Springer Publishing Company, Inc.
536 Broadway
New York, NY 10012-3955

Cover design by Margaret Dunin
Production Editor: Jeanne Libby

97 98 99 00 01 / 5 4 3 2 1

Library of Congress Cataloging-in-Publication Data

Kaplan, Barry Jay.
    A nurse's guide to public speaking / Barry Kaplan.
       p.   cm.
    Includes bibliographical references and index.
    ISBN 0-8261-9590-3
    1. Communication in nursing.   2. Public speaking.   3. Public speaking for women.   I. Title.
    [DNLM: 1. Communication—nurses' instruction.   2. Speech—nurses' instruction.   3. Public Relations—nurses' instruction.   PN 4121 K17n 1997]
RT23.K37   1997
808.5'1'024613–dc21
DNLM/DLC
for Library of Congress   96-53471
                                                  CIP

Printed in the United States of America.

The author would like to thank Barbara Barnum for her support, encouragement, and guidance during the writing of this book.

Contents

Foreword

Speak up! How often did we cringe when we heard those words as children? Or in school, did we dread those required performances in front of the class? Nurses are not immune from that sort of stage fright. Yet in today's health care environment, more and more nurses find themselves in managerial and corporate positions where they must speak up to be effective. Other nurses find themselves dealing with new publics, from community groups, to advertisers, to political and business groups. Yet other nurses are responsible for increased communications with groups in the workplace. With these ever increasing demands for effective communications, many nurses need to update or acquire skills in public speaking.

Barry Jay Kaplan knows this first hand. When I met Barry, he was getting his first dose of nurses and nursing. And he was amazed. He must have asked me a hundred times, ''Why don't people know about nursing? Why don't nurses tell their story?'' This book is Barry's very personal attempt to help nurses tell that story effectively. Barry came to like nurses, and more important, to respect them. Yet from his orientation as a novelist and dramatist, he was always puzzled at our behavior. ''Nursing,'' he told me many times, ''is the world's best kept secret.''

That is changing—perhaps not fast enough—but it is changing. Nurses are finding their voice, and, hopefully, Barry's book will help those voices sound with greater clarity. I recently observed a very contemporary scene where a group of five head nurses made administrative proposals to their corporate board. Every one of these nurses was organized, poised, used the latest audiovisual aids, and presented a compelling argument for the changes she wanted to make on her unit. I couldn't help but admire their ability to make their cases. These talented persuasions did not involve skills taught in any nursing curriculum, yet a lot depended on the effectiveness of the presentations.

Nurses find themselves faced with the need to communicate with all sorts of publics these days, and they need to do it with flair, imagination, and well-couched arguments. Barry doesn't presume to tell nurses what they should say, but he does tell them how to say it with style. And he makes reading about it fun. This book is practical, advising the nurse what to do from the moment he or she is asked to speak, to the postscript moment when he or she is reading those group evaluations.

There are hundreds of small details that make a difference in the outcome of a speech or presentation, things as trivial as avoiding jewelry that clunks against the microphone or learning how to adjust the tempo of your speech. Yet the relatively inexperienced nurse speaker may not even know what questions to ask, what aspects of preparation deserve careful concern. Barry's book is virtually a case map that covers the territory. Barry addresses everything from organizing a speech, to how to address the room and the audience, to exercises to relax before the performance, to the tricks of delivery. Moreover, he does it all with a good humor that makes the book actually enjoyable. Guaranteed, the reader will get a few laughs along the way. Also, you'll enjoy the comments by experienced nurse speakers who contribute occasional wisdom gleaned from their own performances.

Do his suggestions work? I've seen it happen. Barry does workshops for nurses using the techniques he discusses in this book, and the "before" and "after" performances of participants are amazing contrasts. Let's face it, other than the content of a speech, most hints on speaking don't require a brain surgeon to comprehend them. Yet pragmatic as these techniques are, they can make the difference between an audience that offers rousing applause and one that falls asleep in their chairs.

If you are already a speaking pro, don't worry; the book still has much to offer. I learned a lot from it, and I've made more speeches than I should have. Besides, sometimes I need a reminder to do things right, and Barry's book provides that gentle nudge.

Happy reading, and then, happy speaking.

Barbara Barnum, PhD, RN, FAAN
Professor
Columbia University School of Nursing
New York

Introduction

More nurses are speaking in public today than ever before. They are participating in national conferences, panel discussions, seminars and local union meetings, communicating with other nurses and health professionals via telephone and conference calls, leading staff meetings, providing patient education, lecturing to community health leaders, teaching students and peers, acting as management consultants, dealing with social workers, pharmaceutical salespeople, alumnae and professional associations. And as the role of the nurse within the healthcare system changes and grows, the issues on which nurses will communicate via speech will be as broad and various and dynamic as the health industry itself.

We tend to think of public speaking as a formal event, something other people do: professional speakers, politicians, celebrities, people working for a cause, raising money for charity, garnering publicity for a candidate or for the book they've just written. This view of public speaking is accurate but limited. Public speaking, in fact, affects every aspect of oral communication because, at its most basic level, it refers to the ways in which people get ideas and information across, educate people about something they didn't know or persuade them of a particular point of view: all via the spoken word.

And yet it is not as simple as it may seem. There have been times in all our lives when we've been so frustrated at ineffective oral communication that we have had cause to say some of these lines:

"I don't think I'm making myself clear."

"I'm only going to say it one more time."

"You don't understand what I'm talking about."

"Why do I have to keep explaining myself to you?"

Implicit in these remarks is the notion that the fault is in the listener, that they "have not heard you right." While this certainly may be so—listening is a skill in itself—it may also be quite the case that the information has been communicated in a less than effective manner.

While many nurses at every level, staff to manager to executive, complain about the number of papers they have to write—order forms, procedurals, memos—they are called upon to communicate verbally more often and complain about it less. In the daily life of a nurse there are countless times when she has to rely on her speaking abilities to communicate ideas and information: in staff meetings, on the telephone, when explaining complicated procedures to a new nurse, educating patients and families, speaking to doctors, dietitians, lab workers, pharmacists, housekeeping staff, technicians.

Yet many nurses separate lectern-style public speaking from the speaking they do in their many one-on-one meetings. In point of fact, they have a lot in common: Both require preparation, knowledge of the subject matter, clear thinking, and a structured, concise delivery. Both consider who is being spoken to, why the information is being delivered, and how the location affects the presentation. Many of the decisions that go into even the most routine delivery of spoken information are based on a combination of instinct and experience, which together have taught us that it is not enough just to give the information, taking it for granted that the other person will receive it. The information has to be presented in a way that compels the listeners' attention and makes it easy for them to understand and remember just what you want them to.

If the idea of public speaking makes you self-conscious: good. When speaking in public we are naturally more conscious of ourselves than we usually are and that is as it should be. Our voices, our bodies, our gestures all contribute to the effect we want to make, and in order to maximize our potential in these areas we must be aware of how we present ourselves when we speak.

What To Know before You Make Your Speech

1

There are many forms of public speaking we'll consider in this book, including panel discussions, groups discussions, interviews, telephone meetings, and conferences. They have many things in common. But let's begin by taking a look at the hardest case: you behind a lectern, on a podium, making a formal speech to a large group of people. Once you master this, the rest is simple.

Ready?

The president of the head nurses' council you used to belong to calls you at work and asks if you would like to give a talk at the fall members' meeting. The subject: making the transition from union to management. You certainly know the subject, having made just such a transition yourself. You know the pitfalls, the problems, and the rewards, and you've got some humorous anecdotes that would illustrate what you want to say. You're flattered she's thought of you. You check your calendar to see if you're free. You are. "Yes," you say. "I'll be glad to make the speech."

You hang up. Suddenly your hands are sweating and your heart is pounding. You have a vision of yourself standing in the Roman Coliseum, thousands of people looking at you, hands raised, ready to turn thumbs up or thumbs down on what you're about to say—only you're so paralyzed with fear you can't open your mouth.

What have I done, you think. Why did I say yes? I'm unprepared. My throat gets tight when I'm nervous and I'm nervous right now, so how am I going to be when I actually have to give the speech? I don't even know the location where I'll be speaking. I don't know how I let myself agree so readily. I don't know what to wear.

Worst of all, what am I going to say?

Okay. Okay. Calm down. Back up. You're way ahead of yourself. Before you get to composing the speech and deciding whether to wear the black suit or the red dress, there's plenty of preparation you have to do and information you have to get. In fact, you'd better get a pencil and paper and start making a list of questions, then call back the person who offered the invitation to speak. There's a lot you need to ask her.

LOCATION, LOCATION, LOCATION

Knowing as much as you can about where you're going to speak will help you make your speech more effectively. You'll give a different kind of speech, speak in a different way, even use different gestures if you're speaking in a hotel conference room rather than in the training center of a large corporation or a university auditorium, a high school classroom, a gymnasium, a restaurant dining room, or outdoors.

Learn all you can. Assume nothing.

The best thing to do is visit the site. If it's in the town where you live, great. If it's not, it might be worth a short trip. If that's not possible, call your host and have a list of questions ready to ask. Can you get a floor plan of the room? No? Well, then, how big is it? How many people does it seat? Is there going to be a podium? Where is the audience? Are the chairs moveable? Is the floor banked like in a theater? Or is it flat? Is the audience seated around tables, in rows, on folding chairs?

All of these things affect how you will speak, and the fewer surprises, the better you can deal with the situation.

If you can't get to the site to check it out before you speak, the next best thing is to have someone you know and trust check it out for you: a colleague who lives in the town where you'll be giving the speech, someone who has access to the site.

There's a lot to check out beforehand.

You'll probably think of some things yourself. This is a beginning list of questions to ask of yourself, your host, and the technicians involved. Some of the items to follow are within your control: you can change them (or request that someone else change them) or accommodate yourself to them if they can't be changed. Some of the items are not within your power to control or change, in which case it is better to know about them beforehand than to arrive prepared to do one thing and discover that something about the physical properties of the room prevents you from doing it. If you can't get to the site beforehand, you can certainly get there an hour or two before the time you're scheduled to speak. There's plenty for you to do when you arrive.

WINDOWS

Are there any windows? If there are, will the sun be shining in your eyes or in the eyes of your audience? Will your speech be competing with a beautiful view (cherry blossoms blowing in the breeze), a lot of distracting activities (people poolside, people skiing). Can the windows be shaded against such distractions?

LECTERN

Is there a lectern? Does it have a lamp? Is the bulb burned out? What do you do if it is? Is there a shelf under the lectern for your purse, your cough drops, your handkerchief? Is there a lip on the surface that will keep your speech from sliding away? Is the lectern adjustable in terms of height? Failing that, is there a box to stand on?

MICROPHONE

Do you need a microphone? If one is available, does it work? Can you adjust the height? (It should be chin level so it doesn't hide your face and so you don't have to bend over to speak into it.)

LIGHTING

Does the lighting in the room glare in your eyes? Does it glare
in the audience's eyes? Is it bright enough to read by? Is it bright
enough for you to make eye contact with people in the audience?
Is it bright enough for them to read their program and take notes?

SEATING ARRANGEMENTS

Check seating arrangements before the audience arrives. Once
they're seated, they're not getting up. If there are a hundred chairs
spread out all over the room and you know only fifty people are
coming, try to have some of the extra chairs removed and group
the remaining ones close to the center. If the seats are fixed, rope
off the rear area so the audience will be compelled to sit closer
to you.

VENTILATION

Make sure the air conditioning does not make the room too cold
or the heating make it too stuffy. Check and listen for the noise the
temperature controls make. You may want to turn them off for the
duration of your speech or risk competing with a hissing radiator
or a humming cooler.

DOORS

Are the doors at the front and rear of the room? If there are doors
on the same side of the room where you're speaking, make sure
they are locked when you start. Otherwise, you run the risk of
latecomers appearing "on-stage" during your speech.

NOISE

Will other events be going on in adjacent rooms? Find out. Find
out if they're going to be playing music, or batting a ball around,

or cheering. In other words: find out if the rooms are soundproof. Do this by going inside one and listening. Alert the management that you are aware of the potential for noise interference and this should increase their sensitivity to your concerns.

HELP

When you arrive, find out the name and phone number or beeper number of the manager, the maintenance engineer, the sound engineer, or whoever can change a light bulb, adjust the air conditioner, stop a leak, or fix a fuse.

> "I * never accept an invitation unless I know the expectations of the people who have invited me. I listen to them. I ask them questions: What would help you? What are your goals? Why are you inviting me? I then suggest my own ideas. They don't always know exactly what they want so I suggest areas that might be of interest to them. After I tell them my ideas I ask them to think about them for a week and get back to me. During that time I do not necessarily work on the keynote and other addresses but gather information and think of their culture care areas. I prepare what I think fits the group and culture. Then, 3–4 weeks before the conference, I put the ideas all together. By this time, I have a letter of agreement (not necessarily a formal contract) but something that outlines their expectations and what I can do for them—plus my fee. During this time I keep in close touch with them. They may start without knowing the number of participants who will attend except for a rough estimate. I even help them develop their brochure if they ask for help. I often send them a sample brochure. I never assume they know how to bring our joint ideas together into meaningful objectives. What they expect in their evaluations is also discussed."
>
> —Madeleine M. Leininger, PhD, RN, FAAN
> Professor of Nursing and Anthropology,
> Wayne State University, Detroit

---

* The quotes used in *A Nurse's Guide to Public Speaking* all come from interviews with the nurses quoted and are used with their written permission.

KNOW YOUR AUDIENCE

In the course of your work, you wouldn't place a telephone call
and start talking without knowing to whom you were speaking. In
the course of planning a speech, the same basic rules apply: Know
who you're talking to and why you're talking to them.

The person who asked you to speak may not have told you
anything about your audience, or they may have said something so
general it doesn't offer you much help. Saying: "they're all nurses"
or "they're all lab technicians" doesn't go a long way toward
informing you of anything.

There are ways to find out about your audience. The first person
who might be of help is the person who invited you. During your
initial conversation she may simply have neglected to mention what
she knows about the audience, or you may have neglected to ask
for specifics. Now is the time to do that. Call her back and ask. If
she doesn't know, there are other people to ask.

Call and ask the public relations department of the organization
for last year's annual report. If the organization publishes a newsletter, ask the public relations person to send you a copy. What you'll
find out by reading this material are the interests of the organization,
who its officers are, what kind of structure it has. You can also tell
the public relations person who you are and that you'll be speaking
at the next conference. (You might also take advantage of this
opportunity to suggest a little publicity be planned for the upcoming
event.) And ask for any literature (that might be available from the
organization's last conference) that would be helpful to you in
understanding the people to whom you're going to be speaking.

When this literature arrives, read it carefully. With a little investi-
gation, you'll uncover the names of previous speakers. They're
another source. Call and tell them you'll be speaking to the organization they addressed last year. Ask for their reading on the audience.
What did and didn't work? You may even know someone who'll
be in the audience, another good source of information.

Use common sense and your inherent creativity and you'll be
able to learn about your audience. But, before you start asking
questions, decide what you need to know.

"I was once asked to go to a presentation with a group and the subject was empowerment of women. I prepared a speech on community health issues that were mainly led by women and brought a video on the subject. When I got there I was shocked to learn that the audience was a group of legislators from Washington DC and the subject was not empowerment of women but empowerment as a strategy in general. I had to think on my feet, and adapted my speech to a more general audience. By speaking in a more general way I was able to change the focus of the video too from women to community."

—Helen K. Grace, PhD, RN, FAAN
Program Director, W. K. Kellogg Foundation

WHAT DOES THE AUDIENCE KNOW?

Knowing the educational background of a group will tell you a lot about how much they probably already know about the subject you may have in mind. The more sophisticated they are, the more sophisticated your speech will have to be. You don't want to give a speech on basic pain medication to seasoned oncology nurses. Unless, of course, you believe they need it. On the other hand, the very fact that they're sophisticated means you can tell them something you're pretty sure they don't know. If you've uncovered some little known piece of scholarship or have the inside track on a new technique that's just being developed, a group of nurses who consider themselves up on the latest issues in their specialty will be very appreciative of hearing the last word on a cutting-edge technique.

WHY HAS THIS AUDIENCE COME
TO HEAR YOU SPEAK?

In other words, do you have a captive audience, eager to hear what you have to say, regardless of whether or not they agree? Or is attendance mandatory? An audience that has come to hear you speak whether or not they are interested is a tougher crowd to please. You may want to acknowledge this situation right away in your speech: "I know some of you would rather be on the golf course/ski slope/horseback trail right now than have to listen to me, but I think that when I'm finished . . . in exactly twenty minutes, by the way . . . you'll be glad you were here."

DOES THIS AUDIENCE KNOW YOU?

If the audience knows you, is it by name or by reputation? If you've spoken on this subject before or written articles on it, your audience is likely to have opinions about you as soon as they see your name. It helps if you know their expectations. Whether or not you decide to fulfill their expectations is another matter. You may use the fact that you are a known quantity to startle them with some facts or opinions they weren't expecting. Or take them in a different direction than they thought you would go.

> "I presented a very scholarly speech to a group of nurses, not knowing that I had been recommended by a member of the group who had heard me make a humorous presentation on another topic. All through the speech I felt that something was wrong. Only later did I find out they had expected to be entertained more than educated."
>
> —Barbara Stevens Barnum, RN, PhD, FAAN
> Editor of *Nursing Leadership Forum*,
> Consultant, Nursing Division,
> Columbia Presbyterian Medical Center

IS THIS AUDIENCE INTERESTED IN YOU? IN YOUR SUBJECT?

Will the audience be informed beforehand as to the subject of your speech, or will they find out only when they sit down at the event and read the program? How much do they know about the subject? Where did they get this information? How much more do they need or want to know? Does this group have preconceived ideas about you or about your subject? If they do, you may want to reassure them that their perception is safe in your hands. Or, you may want to shake them up by revealing some new or contradictory ideas. Is this audience with you or against you?

If you're going to be speaking to a group of doctors on the role of the nurse practitioner in a rural setting, it helps to know that you may be facing a hostile or suspicious audience. While it can be very soothing to address a roomful of people who already agree with you, it can be an exciting challenge to attempt to convert people who are not on your side to your way of thinking, or at least to open the door for a spirited discussion.

WHO IS THIS AUDIENCE?

Are they pharmaceutical salespeople, medical suppliers, doctors, lawyers, technicians, specialists? If they are other nurses, at what level of education, or of which specialty are they?

HOW MANY PEOPLE WILL ATTEND?

Group dynamics is an interesting phenomenon. The way people behave in groups changes according to many variables. Do they know each other? Do they work together? Do they have similar jobs or the same professional interests? Not so obvious, but equally important, is the way in which the size of a group affects audience behavior.

People in small groups probably know each other and probably will pay closer attention to what you say, basically because it's too risky to daydream. It's likely that someone is going to ask them their opinion. Because they know each other—and are likely to have certain experiences in common—they frequently anticipate each other's reactions to new ideas. You know this is happening when you say something they haven't heard before and all around the room people are turning to look at each other in agreement or disagreement—not necessarily with you, but with each other.

People in large audiences, on the other hand, are more likely to be anonymous both to you and to each other. As a result, they feel less pressure to listen. It's easier to daydream. It is unlikely that anyone is going to quiz them on what they've heard. Therefore, your speech needs to be more dramatic, more entertaining, more inspiring. You need to get them to react by challenging them, startling them, surprising them, getting them to participate by asking questions that make them think.

KNOW THE OCCASION

Here are some of the basic questions you'll want answered.

Why Does This Group Meet?

Is this a regular meeting? Is it a group that convenes every Thursday from 7 to 9? Is it a regular practice of this group to have people come in and speak to them? Do they already know you, either by name, title, or association?

Is This Occasion a Special Event?

Is the occasion a celebration, an anniversary, a sales conference, a seminar, a continuing education lecture?

Is It Formal?

Will the leaders of the organizations be there, which means that everyone is on their best behavior? Or is it for middle management, a group of equals, so that the mood is more casual?

Will Food Be Served?

Is a meal going to be served before you speak? People who've just eaten a big meal tend to stay in a social, casual mood for a while, so if your speech is very serious, you'll need to lighten it up at the beginning to draw them in. Is a meal going to be served *while* you're speaking? This is a tough situation, because your competition is a person's appetite, and if that person is hungry, you're in trouble. If this is the case, it's best to acknowledge the situation good-naturedly rather than pretend it isn't happening.

What about Noise?

Consider that the noise level in the audience will be higher during a meal: the sound of silverware, plateware, and glasses. Expect that at least one of the waiters is going to drop a tray of chicken à la king just when you've reached a climactic moment in your speech. It's best to be prepared for this with a joke: "I didn't expect such an explosive reaction to my speech!"

Will Drinks Be Served?

If alcoholic drinks are served, you can expect to face an audience that is at best relaxed, at worst inattentive.

OTHER THINGS TO KNOW

What Is the Ratio of Men to Women in the Audience?

An audience of male nurses has different interests, different needs, and a different perspective on the role of nurse from those of a female audience.

What Is the Economic Status of the Group?

If the group is known to you to be low paid, this can predict their point of view if you're giving a talk on hospital costs, layoffs, or cutbacks. They may have different needs and different resentments and different values from those of a well-paid audience.

When Will You Be Speaking?

Think about what the time of day means to the audience:

1. *Breakfast:* They had to get up earlier than usual. They still face a whole day of work. Be brief.

2. *Mid-morning/just before lunch:* They've had a tough morning. They're hungry. Avoid a darkened room at this time of the day. Your audience might nod out.

3. *Mid afternoon:* The day is almost over. The 3:00 p.m. blahs are setting in. Try not to be the last speaker of the afternoon. If you are, keep it short and energetic.

4. *Early evening:* Have they just eaten? A full stomach is not conducive to rapt attention. You'll have to be lively or they'll drift.

5. *Late evening:* They've had time to refresh themselves after a day's work, a shower, and a good meal. Take advantage of their good mood, but don't ruin it with a long or overly serious speech.

> "The worst case is when the audience is dozing. Especially after lunch. I once gave a talk in Japan. They wanted the written paper beforehand so they could translate it. The way it worked was that I would speak a paragraph and the translator would then speak it in Japanese. And this was after lunch! The audience just conked out, though I was told that it is not considered rude in Japan to close your eyes and nod during someone's speech."
>
> —Chris Tanner, PhD, RN, FAAN
> Professor, Oregon Health Sciences University,
> School of Nursing, Portland

How Long Do You Have?

People speak at 150 words a minute, so three double-spaced typewritten pages takes five minutes to deliver. Calculate your time. Don't leave it to chance.

Who Else Is Speaking and
What Are They Going To Say?

Ask for a copy of the other speakers' speeches; at least find out the topic of their speech. You certainly don't want to find yourself in the position of following someone who has just said exactly what you're about to say. And, if they've said the opposite of what you're about to say, you want to know about it beforehand so you prepare an appropriate response.

If you can't get advance copies of the speeches, ask for the speakers' telephone numbers. Call and confer with them. You'll all be better off if you know what the other is going to speak about. And the occasion will go better too.

Know the Remunerative Arrangements

Ask if there is a fee involved. Don't be embarrassed to do this. Asking is not demanding. Asking does not mean that you won't accept the invitation if you're not paid. But don't assume that you'll be paid, only to discover later that such was never the organization's intention. Prevent any hard feelings by discussing this up front. Many people will ask you in advance what your fee will be. Be prepared with a figure. Ask friends whom you consider to be comparable to yourself in experience and background what they charge for similar presentations.

If there is no fee for this engagement, you will want to know if the organization provides transportation, a room and meals, or how these items will be arranged. Don't assume that, because you're going to have to travel and spend the night, they're going to pay for it. Ask about the arrangements. Are you expected to lay out the money for everything and submit receipts for reimbursement?

If you're on your own in terms of travel, accommodations, and meals, you may not want to accept the invitation. You'd certainly be within the boundaries of good sense and politeness to say so. You may even indicate that you would be happy to come if they would pay for your expenses.

Should You Speak for No Money?

Certainly you've got something better to do on a Saturday afternoon than get dressed up to stand in front of 500 people with your knees knocking and your palms sweating. On the other hand, do you really have something better to do? Let's assume for the moment that you have decided never to speak in public unless you're paid. It seems like a good decision; after all, you're a professional and you think you are well within your principles to expect to be paid when you are executing a professional task. And then you get an invitation to speak in front of a prestigious group of nurses—the very group whose attention you've been hoping to get. Your initial response is to say ''yes.'' Then you're told that you are expected to speak for no money.

Quick. Is your first response one of disappointment? After all, you've made that personal decision never to speak without getting paid for it. Are you going to have to stick with that position? Or are you going to be able to bend it to suit the occasion? You will have to weigh the advantages of speaking in front of this particular group against your own professional vow.

On the other hand, you may feel that this occasion is worth footing the bills yourself because of what it may do for you, namely, give you a chance to meet significant people in your field, provide the opportunity to present your ideas to an audience that most needs to hear them, and avail yourself of the opportunity for visibility to your peers and the nursing leadership. In fact, the speech may be giving you more than you are giving it.

How Much Should You Charge?

There is probably no such thing as an average fee. What you are paid—if you are paid at all—depends on a variety of factors, including the type and size of the organization and your expertise, visibility, experience, and popularity as a speaker. The range of payment for giving a speech is wide, from highs of $2,000 to lows of absolutely nothing.

> ''My biggest fear about public speaking is not getting paid.''
>
> —Barbara Stevens Barnum

Prepare Your Speech

2

HOW TO START

Sometimes you are sought out as a speaker because of your reputation, or because of an office you hold. When that happens, you may be told to select a topic of your own choice. This sounds ideal, but sometimes it's more difficult than a specific assignment.

The mistake some nurses make in deciding what they're going to speak about is in overlooking the obvious. They think too much about all the topics they might choose, when, in fact, the topic they *should* be talking about is staring them in the face. The first rule of speechmaking is this: *start with what you know*. As a nurse, you've been dealing with patients, families, doctors, social workers, pharmacists, technicians, and administrators for your entire career. You've probably specialized in one or several areas. You've got dozens of ideas about your practice tucked away in your mental file. You don't have to search very far to pick your topic. You already know what you want to say.

Once you've narrowed the possibilities from "anything in the world of nursing" to "anything in the world of nursing that you already know," give yourself the gift of time to think seriously and deeply about what it is you're going to select. Put yourself in a quiet room. Unplug the telephone or turn on the answering machine. Tell your kids to refer all their questions to their dad. Tell your husband not to knock on your door for an hour.

Now, whatever you do, don't write, don't plan, don't organize, and don't worry. Just sit down, lean back, and let your mind wander. Go over what you already know about the subject. When you have a random thought, jot it down. Follow that thought until it leads somewhere interesting or until you come to a dead end with it. By the end of the hour, you should have written down enough to get yourself started. At least you've narrowed the field of possibilities down to two or three.

> "My advice would be to find out who you are and give a speech from that knowledge and position. Speakers need to try on different approaches and see what works, what strategies work best for you, not just adopting the ideas and formats of other speakers."
>
> —Chris Tanner

WHAT DO YOU KNOW AND FEEL ABOUT THIS TOPIC?

Start compiling facts, opinions, and examples. No doubt the hospital or school you're associated with has a terrific library or you can plug into Medline on your computer, so that all the research you could want is easily at hand. For the moment, stay away from the library and turn your computer off. There'll be plenty of time for that later. For now, stick to resources that are even closer at hand.

GO THROUGH YOUR FILES

Look up the articles you've clipped out, the newsletters you've saved, and the notes you've written to yourself in the margins of some of your nursing books. Leaf through magazines related to your subject. Talk to friends and business associates. At the same time, start putting together a list of quotes, some valuable statistics, and a couple of interesting examples that support your point. Call up a specialist in the field and ask for a comment; experts love to demonstrate their expertise, and a comment by one of them lends credibility and sophistication to your speech.

"I have a core group of information that I've prepared over the years of doing speeches. I can pull in information from all my other files, from interesting articles. I only file things that I'm interested in."

—Karlene Kerfoot, PhD, RN, CNAA, FAAN
Senior Vice President, Nursing,
St. Luke's Episcopal Hospital, Houston

LOOK AT YOUR NOTES

See which of them might need to be backed up by statistics (nine out of ten do), beefed up with quotations (to add credibility, to strengthen a point, for humor, for shock, for contemporary relevance, for historical comparison), dramatized using examples (be sure to be fair; it's easy—and off-putting to an audience—to make someone or something look foolish). Highlight your topic with comparisons and contrast (if they can do it, we can do it); clarify your points with definitions. Decide where you need examples, statistics, or backing up by authorities.

GO TO THE LIBRARY

You're bound to find a lot of great stuff. Now you must go through it, pick out the best of it, and throw most of it away. It may represent the fruits of your labor; all the information you've gathered may contain a fascinating detail, a shocking statistic, a scandalous opinion but, if it is not relevant to your speech, it has to go. Of course, it may go only as far as your file, perhaps to be used another day in another speech. But unless it advances your point or illustrates your thesis, be ruthless: let it go. You'll also want to leave out anything that is unverifiable, no matter how gripping or astounding, and anything you suspect might come back to haunt you. (Imagine it being broadcast on the late news; imagine your mother showing you a clipping of it a year from now and ask yourself if you would be proud of it or regretful.)

PICTURE YOUR AUDIENCE
WHEN DOING YOUR RESEARCH

Since your speech is an attempt to communicate with them, it is essential that you consider your subject from the audience's point of view as well as from your own. This doesn't mean that you will cater to the audience or alter your own thoughts to pander to what you perceive are theirs. It does mean that you want to make sure you are making clear exactly how the information you're presenting pertains to their concerns. Will the information earn them money? Will it save them time? Does it promote their health and longevity? Does it increase their understanding of a particular medical or social issue? Will it increase their satisfaction in their work? Will it offer a new perspective on something in which they had been entrenched?

> "I use examples that are personal to the audience. Then I know I've captured them. If I see some are nodding out, I try to speak to them directly. If I know the audience, I use individuals as examples of what I'm talking about."
>
> —Linda S. Hurwitz, RN, MA
> Vice President for Nursing,
> Babies and Childrens Hospital,
> Columbia Presbyterian Medical Center, New York

WRITING THE SPEECH

Here's a startling fact: It is impossible just to sit down and write a speech. Just as any medical procedure is done one step at a time, so is a speech written, one step at a time. If you think of speech writing in this way, you will never be faced with the admittedly daunting prospect of writing the speech. With all the research and thinking you've put in so far, you've already done half the work when you actually sit down to write.

Compose one concise sentence that clearly states your purpose. This is something you can refer to whenever you find yourself unsure as to how to proceed. If your purpose is clear, you will always be able to find your way.

The Opening

In the opening you tell them what you're going to tell them: "I'm here today to talk about the social injustice and economic waste that occur when older nurses are forced into early retirement."

Grab their attention at the beginning and you're halfway home. Lose them at the beginning and it's uphill all the way.

Don't flash a phony smile and tell them how nice it is to be there or show false enthusiasm in saying what a wonderful group they are or what an honor/pleasure/thrill it is to speak to them. These kinds of flowery, excessive opening lines are a waste of time, not individualistic, and who believes them anyway? As phrases go, they're so overused they don't mean anything. If you must say you're glad to be there, tell them why.

Don't apologize. If you're late or unprepared or your slides were in luggage that got lost by the airline or someone spilled a glass of cranberry juice on your white linen suit, give a simple and brief explanation of what happened and get on with your speech. Unless you plan to call off the speech, don't indulge in long-winded excuses.

Let the audience know you know who they are. If they're nurses at an urban hospital that's just undergone budgets cuts and layoff, express sympathetic understanding. If they're nurse practitioners, bristling from having been labeled as "physician extenders" by their CEO, let them know you applaud their efforts to change his perspective. Show that you identify with their goals and principles.

Pose a provocative question that leads into the body of your speech. Make the people in the audience think about their own answer. Set up expectations that your speech will either meet or confound.

State an amazing fact to introduce your subject. "Last year, the number of employed nurses over the age of 55 fell by 35 percent. This is twice the national average for men of any profession over the age of 55, and three times that of women in other professions."

Let the audience in on something about your own life that reflects your subject. Perhaps your professional credits or experiences will let you illustrate why you are the best person to give the speech you're about to give.

Humor is a category in itself and is sometimes no laughing matter, especially if you try a joke and get no response. Then the audience is embarrassed and you're starting from behind. On the other hand, there is nothing that will get an audience's attention and enthusiasm more effectively than a good laugh. Remember, there is nothing that loses an audience more quickly than a joke that isn't funny, so proceed at your own risk. But remember that once a joke has worked, it'll probably work again.

The Body

In the body of your speech you must support your thesis with facts, quotations, and statistics.

Organize your thoughts. Refer back to that one sentence that clearly states your purpose, and you'll realize that, although you may have a lot to say, you can't say it all and shouldn't even try. Remember that the audience is listening to you, not reading your words in a book, in which case they would have time to reflect, to go back, to take a break, to proceed at their own pace, to reread something they didn't quite understand. When they're only listening to you speak, the number of points you can make must be limited.

Your material—a combination of research, quotations, statistics, opinions—must be focused around your central idea. Once that idea is made clear to you and to your audience, you can branch off and make a few other points. But you'll always relate them back to the main point. Organizing those thoughts into a coherent whole, one that flows logically from one idea to the next, can be accomplished in several different progressions.

Organize by time. Show how your subject was once, the stages it went through, and the place it is now. In other words, start with the past and go step-by-step into the present and end by suggesting what the future holds. Of course, you will want to make the audience see how the past, present, and future you're describing affect their lives. "If the rate of nursing layoffs of the past continues, your future, when you're older, holds a grim picture."

Organize by influence. Demonstrate how one thing affects another: how nursing education affects bedside nursing, for example.

You may even begin by identifying how lack of a certain kind of education can lead to an unfortunate experience, perhaps one of your own. The personal admission is very effective when presenting information, because it not only takes the idea out of the theoretical and into the real, but also because the audience will sympathize with the honesty of your admission.

Organize by sequence. You can use numbers to give a form to your subject: "There are seven things every nurse has to know in order to keep her job past the age of 55." Then you go on to delineate them, one by one.

Organize by problems and solutions. With this progression you begin by identifying a problem: "Older nurses are losing their jobs at an alarming rate." Then you present all the problems and explain the ways in which they play themselves out. Use statistics, headlines, and personal experiences. Next, you offer a solution or several solutions. Don't underestimate the audience's intelligence by pretending the solution will be easy if, in fact, it will be difficult. If there is a sense of crisis to the problem as you see it, identify it as such, but don't be an alarmist. Later, you won't want to be thought of as the nurse who cried wolf.

Organize by location. You may organize your argument by showing how the trend of older nurse layoffs progresses as you move eastward across the country. Or south from the north. Can trends be spotted? Can sense be made of the statistical differences geographically?

Organize by the ABC's. A long list of items, with no one of them being more or less important than any other, can be organized according to the alphabet. It's a simple progression and it always works to keep the audience focused and on track. It's also a way to use humor as you go. And it's very versatile; you don't have to worry about finding a sentence that begins with every single letter. "**A** is for **all** the reasons older nurses are forced into early retirement." The same sentence slightly reworked can also work this way: "**F** is for the reasons older nurses are **forced** into retirement." In other words, you can make the alphabet serve you in many ways.

Organize by acronym. An alternate to the ABC route is to construct a convenient acronym. For example: **SACRED: S**implified **A**dditions to the **C**onstruction of **R**ehabilitation and **E**ducation **De**partments.

Vocabulary

Choose your words carefully. The spoken word has properties different from the written word. A listening audience's comprehension is different from a reader's, just as a person's spoken vocabulary is smaller than a person's reading vocabulary. This means that what is appropriate on the page, where the reader has the time to look as long as she likes, may not be appropriate or even comprehensible when spoken on the stage, where the words go by in an instant.

Your goal is to communicate, not to demonstrate that you can wrap your mouth around a six-syllable word. An audience is most impressed with the speaker who makes herself clear, so keep it simple: use words that are to the point and appropriate to your audience and to your subject.

Practice Aloud

Do you feel comfortable saying these words? If you don't, what are the chances of making the audience comfortable in hearing them?

Stay Away from Slang

Steer clear of slang, shorthand, euphemisms, unexplained acronyms, verbs used as nouns, nouns used as verbs, and especially any language that would not be understood by people outside of a special interest group.

Avoid Hyperbole

Don't try to pump up the importance of what you're saying by using words like "great," "extremely," and "very." Instead, use examples of your subject's greatness. Saying that Martha Rogers is a great writer is not as dramatic as quoting her or citing her publications and the influence they have had on the profession.

Foreign Expressions

There are three cardinal rules concerning foreign words:

1. Make sure your pronunciation is correct;

2. Choose only foreign words appropriate to your subject;
3. Be sure that your audience understands them.

To be on the safe side, you could say: "The French have a word for it," or "only the Germans have an expression that describes this."

Sexist Language

Avoid sexism. Nurses are used to referring to nurses as "she" because most nurses are women. You won't always be talking to or about nurses, however, and you'd be better off using something more neutral like "he or she." Often this is clumsy in spoken speech, so you might want to shift to the plural: Instead of "he or she does his or her work," try "they do their work."

Unusual Words

Don't assume your audience knows everything. On the other hand, don't offend them by spoon-feeding them things they probably do know If, in making a particular point, it is important that your audience's definition of a word is in precise agreement with your own, there's nothing wrong with introducing it by saying: "According to the Random House Dictionary . . . " This doesn't offend anyone by assuming their ignorance, and is a way of making sure you and they are cued in to the particular subtleties of the word's meanings. Reading aloud the dictionary definition might even be used to set up the fact that you and the audience may be using the term differently.

Statistics

Make statistics fascinating. Numbers can be very impressive when written in a paper and read by someone at leisure. But that same list of numbers that dazzles the eye is apt to bore an audience. There are several ways to make statistics vital and memorable. First, relate the numbers to the concerns of the audience: "Over the course of the next year, five thousand nurses will lose their jobs. Will you be one of them?'' Second, make the numbers you use memorable: ''Nearly half a million nurses suffer stress-related accidents every year,'' instead of ''483,567 nurses.'' Third, give the numbers a graphic image: Instead of ''emergency room visits are increasing at the rate of four a day nationally,'' say: ''If you took all of last year's additional ER patients and put them together, there'd be enough people to keep all the physicians in the state of Vermont busy for a year.''

Quotations

Use quotations effectively. Use them with variety: from Franklin Roosevelt, John Kennedy, Walt Whitman, Socrates, Hippocrates, Dorothea Dix, the vice president of nursing of the local hospital to the President of JCAHO. Keep quotes simple and to the point. Buy a copy of *Bartlett's Familiar Quotations*, where quotes are found by subject, author, and first line. Use quotes sparingly. Too many brilliant and witty quotes from other people and your audience will begin to wonder why you're the one speaking instead of the people you're quoting. Make quotations seamless with your own words, and make them back up your own words. Set them up as contrast to your own words, and make sure you know how to pronounce the source's name correctly.

> ''When I put a speech together I pull from my files all the salient points from articles and write my opinions with backup and quotes. I have a quote file in my word processor, filed according to topic. I also use *The Manager's Book of Quotations* by Lewis Eigen and Jonathan Siegal (American Management Association, 1989). Once I've got the content, I use the quotes to spice things up.''
>
> —Karlene Kerfoot

> ''I usually start only my keynote with a scholarly quote from nurse scholars or others such as Plato. Then I'll say something like: 'Today more than ever before nursing has great opportunities.' I develop my challenges and focus on the purpose and intent of my address.''
>
> —Madeleine Leininger

Other Tips

- Short sentences are stronger than long sentences. In addition, you don't run the risk of getting out of breath before you come to the end of a thought. If you think the sentence is too long, it probably is. Cut it.
- The active voice is stronger than the passive voice.
- Expressions such as ''I think,'' ''I believe,'' ''In my opinion,'' actually make your point weaker. If you are speaking and you don't attribute the thought or opinion to anyone else, the audience knows you think it, you believe it, and it is your opinion.
- Resist this temptation to qualify what you're going to say. Just say what you want to say. Cut to the chase.

The Closing

In closing, you tell them what you just told them: ''And so we've seen the many ways and the reasons why nurses are forced to retire before they are ready.''

Here's your chance to sum up all your important points. It's not the time to put forth any new thoughts. Remember that your conclusion is the last thing your audience will hear. Give it all you've got. Here are some methods to close your speech in a compelling way.

A Personal Story

Dramatize how everything you've been talking about came together in a personal way.

The Big Picture

Relate how the points you've made fit into the larger picture of health care or nursing, in general, or your regional hospital.

A Rhetorical Question

"If we want to preserve our right to hold our jobs past the age when most nurses are being forced to retire, do we dare to take the risk and do what I'm suggesting? The real question is: dare we take the risk and do nothing?"

THE KISS PRINCIPLE OF STYLE:
KEEP IT SHORT AND SIMPLE

"If I don't know the material well I make an outline first, then actually write the speech, then read it. I write it in the way I talk, not so it sounds like a formal speech. I make side comments to myself in the margin, reminding myself to give an example. This way I can make sure to cover all the points and also be spontaneous."

—Linda S. Hurwitz

The Manuscript

Once you've written your speech, you want to prepare the physical manuscript in a way that will make it easy for you to speak from it. Simply typing the speech neatly, in the form you would type a manuscript to submit for publication will not serve you best. Here are some things you can do to make the speech easier to read.

- Write large enough to read in dim light without glasses. If you've typed your speech on a computer, you may want to print it out in **bold**, ALL UPPER CASE, *italics*, or in a larger type size than normal.
- Use a red pencil to mark cues to visual aids, moments to pause for dramatic effect, when you're going to look up and make eye contact with the audience.
- Double-space between lines.
- Triple-space between paragraphs.
- Don't hyphenate words at the end of a line.
- Don't break statistics at the end of a line.

- Don't break a sentence on a page.
- Write out abbreviations.
- Spell out foreign names or difficult medical phrases phonetically.
- Use ellipses . . . to indicate where you will pause.
- Bind the pages so they don't slip from your grasp, but keep them loose enough so that it will be easy to lay them out flat.
- Don't use paper that is so slick it is difficult to turn the pages.
- Make two copies and keep each in a different place. Don't pack both in your suitcase. What if the airline loses your luggage?

> "I usually make an outline. 85% of the time I turn this into overheads and speak from selected words. The overheads are clear and simple. I have a copy in front of me with notes on the bullets. I never speak from a formal text. If I have to submit a paper, I write it out first then do an abstract of it later."
>
> —William L. Holzemer, PhD, RN, FAAN
> Professor, University of California–San Francisco

> "I type out the titles of the slides. Then I write the kinds of things I want to talk about, just notes to make me remember, usually in handwriting. Only once or twice have I spoken from a written text because if I have to read a speech, I'm dead in the water. I like to liven up my speeches with chit chat."
>
> —Karlene Kerfoot

Visual Aids

A speech is more than words. Just as every gesture you make, every tilt of your head or toss of your wrist, every shrug, or nod, or raised eyebrow, adds to—or subtracts from—your message, so, too, do all the visual aids you select. There's a vast array from which to choose, ranging from a complete synchronized sound film or video to a sophisticated, professionally produced color slide presentation, to typewritten overheads to handmade posters written while you speak, in front of the audience. Whatever visual aids you select, they can serve as valuable ways to anchor your speech and as reinforcement of your points for the audience. No matter which you use, there are certain principles that are worth paying attention to:

- Tell the audience what they're going to see, then show it to them.
- Keep charts simple.
- Use bold colors, a dark background, and light type.
- Make sure everyone in the room can see clearly. (Don't stand in your own way.)
- Illustrate only what's hard to visualize.
- Don't use the visuals to echo your words.
- Show what's essential. Avoid small details.
- Only illustrate key points of your speech.

Slides

- Use one slide for one point.
- Use slides only if they contribute new information or help the audience understand what you're saying.
- Don't use them if they complicate the issue, take away from what you're saying, or if you're using them to help you through a spot in the speech that you haven't clearly thought out.
- Avoid abbreviations.
- Use simple sentences.
- Make sure the ideas in one slide follow a logical order.
- Use Upper and lower case letters, NOT ALL CAPS.
- Use a screen, not a wall or curtain.
- Talk to your audience, not your display.
- Before the meeting, check to see how your slides look from the back of the room and the sides of the room.
- Read the slide slowly to yourself to determine how long the slide has to stay on the screen in order for everyone to read it.
- Remember that slides need a darkened room. Arrange for an assistant to control the lighting. Also, consider how long you want the audience's attention away from you and on the slides.

Don't forget that you are just a disembodied voice during this part of the speech.

Overheads

- Attractive overhead transparencies usually can be seen without turning off the lights, which is a distinct advantage over slides. But you'll need someone to tend to the mechanics. As with slides, be very sure that they are all in the correct order and that the assistant doesn't inadvertently put them on the reverse side.
- Two other advantages of overheads: they are relatively inexpensive and they can be altered with a marker pen.

Videotape

- Check to make sure that your tape fits the available system. Test it ahead. If your tape is on VHS, for example, make sure the VCR is not in BETA format. If your tape is half-inch, make sure the VCR is not three-quarter inch.
- Find out how many monitors are available and be certain each works. Make sure they are in focus and that the speakers enable everyone to hear. Adjust the volume before you begin your speech. Make arrangements for the tape to be turned on, ideally, by an assistant.

Flip Charts

- Maximize the boldness of their graphic appeal.
- If you're using a graph, make sure it's clear.
- Use only a few lines.
- Use different colors to differentiate between chart movements or curves.

Chalkboard

- Don't use it if you have to turn your back too often.
- Don't use it if your handwriting or printing isn't clear.

- Only use it if spontaneity is what's needed in your talk.
- Have a box of spare chalk handy.

> "With the new computers, you can print out your overheads in a reduced size, 8 to a page. I use these as handouts for the audience to follow what I'm talking about. Otherwise I find that they spend all their time copying the overheads and don't listen to me."
>
> —William L. Holzemer

> "I never give out my speech in advance as I want them to listen anew to what I have to say. I may give them a page of concepts, models, or questions for the conference packet, but I want them to listen to my address. I do not want them to be reading while I'm talking."
>
> —Madeleine Leininger

Prepare Yourself

3

PRACTICE THE SPEECH

Don't expect to be satisfied the first time you do it. That is why it is called practicing. You rehearse the speech until you feel comfortable doing it. Don't expect too much from yourself the first few times. Your initial goal is to become familiar with the material and to notice what areas you have difficulty in saying aloud.

You can practice alone in your room, but not slumped in a chair or lounging on a bed. Try to recreate the kind of physical circumstances in which you'll actually be speaking.

Be aware of sentences that go on so long you don't have time to take a breath. Watch for words that make you stumble, or phrases that sound forced, stilted, or pretentious when you speak them aloud. (There may be words that you feel comfortable writing, but feel uncomfortable in saying aloud. Your speech should sound like someone speaking, not like someone reading a paper.)

Become familiar enough with the speech that you are not overly dependent on the written speech when you deliver it. Be aware of how often you refer to the written paper. You don't want to bob your head up and down during your speech, nor do you want to go so long without looking at it that when you finally do you've lost your place.

Stages of Preparation

Practice makes perfect. As a general rule of thumb, you should rehearse about one hour for every minute of your speech. Try giving the speech with a stopwatch in your hand. If you've been given ten minutes to speak and your speech runs fifteen minutes long, practice time is the time to cut it. (When you actually make the speech, bring a watch or small clock with you and set it on the podium so you can see it. This will help you keep to the time that's been allotted. You wouldn't want the speaker before you to take up some of your time, you don't want to take up any of the time of the speaker who comes after you.)

> "I once ran into a situation in which the speaker before me took up her own time and half my time. I was already angry when I began speaking. The way I coped was to shorten my speech. I gave the key points but I wanted to make sure that I finished on time. I got a big hand at the end for doing that. I could tell the audience was afraid that I was going to take all my time and that would have kept them there longer. In situations like this you have to take responsibility to care for the audience. They love you for it."
>
> —Linda S. Hurwitz

Try giving the speech into a tape recorder. Play it back and listen to yourself objectively. We never sound the way we think we do, and once you get over the initial jolt of how you sound, pay critical attention. Check to see that you can be understood, that you don't slur your words, that you're not speaking too fast or too slow, that your pace is varied, that your pauses have the desired effect of emphasizing what you've said, that your speech isn't peppered with "you know" and "uh," and that your voice doesn't rise to a question at the end of a statement.

Should you also do a videotape of yourself? There is a good deal of disagreement on this point. On the one hand, videotaping yourself allows you the opportunity to critique not just your tone of voice, but also all your physical mannerisms. The reasons for the contro-versy are that people are often made overly self-conscious by looking at themselves in the unforgiving light of a TV camera. In addition, the impact a person makes physically on an audience is very different from the impact she makes on a television camera. In other words, videotaping your speech is probably most useful if you are eventually going to give your speech on television.

Prepare Your Voice

The female voice is naturally pitched higher than the male voice, but many women cling to the voice they had as a twelve-year-old, which is higher than their natural voice. A little girl's voice is definitely not authoritative. It does not carry the signs of power or strength, knowledge, or expertise, leadership, or experience. Often the woman with the little girl's voice is educated, experienced, knowledgeable, and strong. She may not even be aware of the shortcoming in her voice. Often the voice is no more than an unfortunate holdover from the past. There is no reason why such a woman should not overcome this. Here are some ways to do it.

Breathe deeply. Use your breath to push the sound from behind. Little-girl voices often let the sound ride on breath. The voice is breathy and light.

Bring your pitch down. Your natural voice is probably lower than the voice you're using. To find your natural voice, put your hands over your ears and start humming at the top of the scale and move slowly down. The point of greatest reverberation is your actual correct pitch.

Speak from your chest. Keep a hand on your chest when you speak. This will remind you to think lower, so, instead of speaking from a constricted throat, you place your voice lower in your chest. Feel the vibrations your voice makes.

Other vocal problems. Huskiness, harshness, hoarseness: we lump these terms together to describe pushing-from-the-throat voice production. This comes as a result of confusing forceful personality with vocal force. Shrillness and stridency, pressuring the pitch upward . . . such voices come out low and gravelly or high and shrieky . . . both are hard on speakers' throats and listeners' ears. This kind of extreme pushed quality can be seen as well as heard: veins on the neck stand out, faces flush with effort. All this comes from constriction in the low and high throat areas, stiffness in the tongue and lips, and tightness in the jaw. The result is likely to be recurrent bouts with laryngitis. The following techniques will bring relief to an aching neck and throat and ease the pushed voice.

- Massage the face and throat. Let your jaw sag. Stroke your throat with your fingertips.
- Stick out your tongue. Don't force it out or thrust it out. Do it five times.
- Ease your jaw. With hands on both sides of your chin, move your jaw from side to side. Let your hands do it. Again, let your hands move your chin up and down.
- Soften your neck. Use your fingers to find the small muscles in the front of your neck that move when you swallow. Massage them gently.
- Loosen the back of your neck. Raise your head up and let it fall down. Repeat several times. Then shake your head very slowly from side to side.

> "I noticed especially when I talked on TV that I talked very quietly and didn't flex my voice. I learned that I had to speak up. What I did was mimic people who spoke on TV all the time. I recorded Jane Pauley, listened to her and imitated her inflections. When you play a recording of this new way of speaking, you sound fake to yourself but it sounds good: not as good as Jane Pauley but better than I sounded before. It's good to have more inflection, range and variety."
>
> —Karlene Kerfoot

Prepare Your Appearance

What you look like should not be as important as what you say, so you don't want to make a bold fashion statement that detracts from or distorts your message. Wear something you feel comfortable in, which people have told you in the past makes you look good. Consider appropriateness; don't dress too casually or too formally. If you try it on and think it might be too flashy, follow that hunch and wear something more conservative. Women should carefully consider hemline length and heel height; men should consider sock height and sleeve length (you want to avoid showing ankles and wrists). Keep your pockets free of anything that might bulge or jangle (keys, coins, bills, notes, pens); keep jewelry to a minimum and keep it small; you don't want your speech to be interrupted by a jangling bracelet only to discover it's on your own wrist. Earrings that dangle may catch the lights, making you look like a blinking Christmas tree to your audience. That hat that looks so good close up may put your face in a shadow, so the audience never sees your expression and never catches your eye. That chic black-and-white checked suit may produce psychedelic effects after the audience stares at it for a while. And materials that rustle will compete with your voice for the microphone.

> "You must be very sensitive to the audience in deciding what to wear. I certainly would dress differently when speaking to a grass roots community organization than I would to a very prestigious leadership conference."
>
> —Helen K. Grace

Last-Minute Checklist

- Remind yourself of all the ways in which you've prepared.
- Reminding yourself how well you've prepared will keep you from worrying about details that you've already taken care of, and help you maintain your confidence. You've left nothing out. You've found out as much as you can before going to make the speech. You've written the speech as carefully and thoughtfully as you can. You've planned your visual aids and executed them with care. You've planned for what to do if things go wrong. You've practiced your speech.
- Remember to prepare an outline of your titles, objectives, and summary description to give to the meeting planners. If CEUs are sought, you may need to provide more details.
- Be sure to make copies of the speech to hand out afterward, if this is appropriate. Always provide a bibliography too.

- Write your own introduction. Even if you mail it ahead, bring along a copy just to be safe. Don't rely on a curriculum vitae. The person introducing you might pick out the wrong items.
- Determine how you'll get to the meeting. If you're driving, get accurate directions and check them on a road map. Fill the car with gas the night before. In case something happens to your car, have the number of a car rental agency and two cab companies ready. Know the train, bus, and plane schedules.
- Pack your glasses, nasal spray, aspirin, contact lens solution, extra pen, spare set of notes, powder to absorb facial perspiration, handkerchief, copies of speech, outline, introduction, and a handful of business cards.
- Check your watch so that you arrive on time.
- However you go, get there early.

BEFORE THE MEETING

It's a month before your speech. You've already checked with the person who invited you and found out all about the audience and the room in which you're going to speak. There remain just a few more details to address before the day on which you'll speak.

Communicate with Meeting Planners

- Give them an outline of your presentation.
- Provide them with your visual aid materials, or let them know what hardware you'll need (projectors, screens, video monitors, etc.). Don't forget to tell them your microphone requirements.
- Give them your introduction.
- Determine if there will be a question-and-answer period after you speak.

> "When I come in to give the keynote speech or workshop I usually arrive the night before. I meet the conference leaders and usually have coffee or dinner with them. As I listen to them I learn more of their interests and needs. The context for my speech is important

as well as to weave their ideas and interest into the talk. Sometimes I revise my talk after listening to the needs of the conference planners—even if at midnight!''

—Madeleine M. Leininger

It's an hour before your speech. You're as prepared as you know how to be. Now that you're on the site where you'll speak, there are a few last-minute details to deal with.

Check the Physical Layout

- Walk around the room.
- Stand at the podium.
- Check its height.
- Make sure there is a place for your notes.
- Check that there is enough light to read them by.

Check the Equipment

- Is the microphone a fixed floor model on an adjustable stand, a console model, or a portable body mike? Test it for height and volume control and see how close you have to be in order to be heard.
- Test the slide projector and the remote control device if it has one.
- Make sure your slides are in the right order.
- Are your tripod, flip chart, and chalkboard set up and ready to go?
- Check that the pointer is within easy reach.

It's ten minutes before you're scheduled to speak. You're breathing deeply, and are as relaxed as a person who is about to speak in public can be (see Relaxation techniques, pp. 33, 44).

Find Out Where You're Supposed To Be Right before You Speak

- Backstage?
- In the audience?
- At the dais?

BEFORE YOU GO ON

Contrary to what you may be thinking, the speech does not begin when you start to speak, but when the audience first sees you, which may be in the lobby of the hotel, the anteroom of the hall where you'll be speaking, when you enter the room, when you're sitting on a raised platform with other panelists or speakers, standing to one side, or at the moment your name is announced and you walk on stage. Your appearance begins the speech. Make sure you're in control of it.

No matter how nervous you are, if there are other speakers before you, pay attention to them. Not only does this make you appear alert and present, these other speakers may even say something that pertains to what you're about to say. Not to have noticed it will not reflect well on you.

Once you've been introduced, all eyes are on you. This is not the time for final touch-ups to your appearance. Check your hair, jewelry, makeup, clothes, and stockings before you appear in front of the audience.

When you go to the podium, carry the speech with you in a neat folder. You don't need to pretend you don't have papers, but you do want to make them look attractive. A mess of loose sheets in your hand does not inspire confidence in your listeners.

Before you begin to speak, take a moment to set yourself up and to do a final check on all the physical elements that involve you. It is better to do this now, before you start, than to start speaking and have something go wrong. Spread out your speech in a way that is comfortable for you. Take a sip of water. Look at the lights. Look at the audience. Ground yourself. Take a deep breath . . .

Wait a second! Before you start speaking, there's something we haven't dealt with.

Fear.
   Nerves.
      Anxiety.
         Aaaaaaaaa!

Breaking the Fear Barrier

4

Public speaking is not an innate skill. Effective public speakers are *made*, through research, observation, hard work, and practice. Giving a speech is not a natural or ordinary event. Most of us, given the occasion to speak in front of a large group of people, would simply prefer not to do so. Speakers who expect to feel at ease are asking for more from themselves than they are likely to be able to deliver. In fact, even the most experienced speakers don't expect to feel relaxed. What you should expect is the nervous excitement and energy that come from the task at hand. You needn't pretend you're not nervous. Instead, confront your anxiety, harness its energy, and use it to your advantage. Here's how.

ADMIT YOUR FEAR

Accept the fact that you're nervous and that it's natural. In fact, it's more natural than not being nervous when standing up in front of a group of strangers. Everyone who gets up in front of groups of people is nervous. The great actor Laurence Olivier had such bad stage fright that he thought he would never be able to act on a stage again and this was after he had already scored his major theatrical successes.

RECOGNIZE THAT FEAR IS NORMAL
FOR PUBLIC SPEAKERS

Who isn't nervous when about to make a speech? No one. Nerves are as common as table salt but a lot harder to shake. Uncontrolled nerves will wreck your speech. Get a grip on them and you can convert your nervousness into useful excitement and energy. In other words, you can use your nerves rather than letting your nerves use you.

> "I'm never relaxed before I speak. As the introduction is being made my mind is racing: will I be OK? I always have a sense of stagefright but I've taught myself that stress is positive. It makes me sharp and alert. I've given some of my worst speeches when I'm not stressed. Once I was out of town to make a speech and when I went to pull the slides, they weren't there! I about died. I had nothing to talk from. My secretary FAXed the notes from the slides but I was so anxious. As it turned out, I was much better than if I'd relied on my slides. I had to project my voice, tell funny stories, really get the audience because I didn't have slides to rely on. That's why I hate slides."

> —Karlene Kerfoot

REALIZE THAT YOUR FEAR
DOESN'T HAVE TO SHOW

You don't have to reveal your nervousness to anyone, not to the person who invited you to speak, not to the other speakers, not to the audience. You can keep it to yourself. You gain nothing by letting others know you're anxious. As a matter of fact, one of the great secrets in conquering fear is this: behave as if you are confident, and you'll begin to feel confident.

VISUALIZE YOURSELF
AS A POWERFUL SPEAKER

If you keep denying your own possibilities—"I'm a terrible speaker and I'll never be able to get up in front of even a small group of people and talk''—you will no doubt stay exactly where you are: afraid. If, on the other hand, you encourage yourself by seeing success in your future—''I can picture myself getting up there in front of everyone and telling them something important''— you have an image of yourself, which, when projected, will be both satisfying and gratifying.

One of the ways that athletes are trained psychologically is that they are asked by their coaches to form a mental image of the thing they're going to do. A ski jumper will close her eyes and envision every step of the way she will make the jump. During the recent Olympics, the figure skaters talked about how they trained even when they weren't on the ice: by going through their program in their minds, picturing how they would do it, how they would look, how it would feel.

Creative visualization can be a very powerful tool in getting you through your speeches. If you've gone over the speech aloud at home, decided just how you want to appear, planned your visual aids, then the only thing you haven't done is the actual speech. But if you take yourself through it, step by step, in your mind, then when you actually do make the speech, the whole process will seem familiar because, in a way, you've already done it.

And, since it's your own imagination, you can imagine the best: that you're in total control, that you look great and feel confident, that you're charming, warm, and enthusiastic, that you're getting a positive audience reaction. Picture yourself hitting all the right notes. Envision the role you want to play and act the part.

Of course, there is a part of you that is nervous and not at all confident, but you gain nothing by dwelling on it. You want to believe in your confident side—the side that is well prepared to give a successful speech.

> ''One thing that helped me was being a camp nurse. Kids want to be entertained and you can't be embarrassed of speaking or leading them. You must act the role. That's what public speaking is: acting the role of a confident speaker.''
>
> —Linda S. Hurwitz

SEE THE AUDIENCE AS YOUR ALLY

Does the audience loom up like some hydra-headed monster, teeth bared? Actually, audiences are nicer than people and they're easier to talk to as well. They won't talk back or challenge you at every turn, at least not until the question period, and by that time you've had your say. Besides, there's the nice attentive hush before you start. Can you count on that in a living room or in the office lounge?

Take the audience into your confidences. If sometimes the right word doesn't come, why not just wonder out loud what it might be? "What's that round thing called when the nurse runs an IV line? I can't think of the word." And someone out of a roomful of nurses will surely call out the answer. Thank them, smile, and bow. The audience will appreciate the levity and spontaneity of the moment.

Many speakers are afraid of the audience. But, if you think about yourself as an audience member, you will see that the audience is not out to get you. An audience wants you to do well. People in an audience are grateful that it's you up there and not them, and they want to show their appreciation.

> "There's always some anxiety no matter how long you've been doing this. I think it can be good, energizing stage fright. My fears leave me once I know that I've gotten to the point where the audience gets what I'm talking about. They may start out with their arms folded across their chests, waiting to see what you're going to say, but at some point they warm up and you know you have them."
>
> —William L. Holzemer

One thing you can do to help you get over fear is to focus on the audience. Identify with your listeners; know as much about them as you can. And remember why you're there: to tell them something in which they're going to be interested. Concentrate on the telling rather than on how nervous you feel. In other words: stop thinking about yourself and think about them. And remember who the expert is. If they knew more than you about this subject, *they* would be giving the speech.

> "I have a trick for quieting my nerves which is to remind myself that the audience is here to be entertained, stimulated and to learn. The main thing to remember is that the group wants to like you. They want to walk away saying: 'that was great!' The fear, of course, is that you are not prepared and the audience will feel they have wasted their time."
>
> —Linda S. Hurwitz

> "A shift I made was to become less concerned with how I looked and more so with the audience learning and getting something out of my speech. It is a matter of getting off yourself. People are there because they want to be. Your aim is to make the best use of their precious time."
>
> —Christine Tanner

SPEAK RATIONALLY TO YOURSELF

Remind yourself that you know what you're talking about (even if it's only knowing how to ask the right questions). Believe in what you're saying (even if it's to say you don't believe something).

> "I'm OK as long as I know the subject. My fears are in not being knowledgeable or when I misread the audience. I'm dependent on audience cues. The worst experience is when I'm not connecting with the audience. My biggest fear is that I'll be going down an entirely different path than the audience. I'll try to reach for examples or illustrations that will bridge this gap. I'm also fearful that I might inadvertently offend the audience by being misinterpreted by them."
>
> —Helen K. Grace

PRACTICE THE SPEECH
USING ALL YOUR VISUAL AIDS

It bears repeating that the more sure you are of your material and all the physical props you've planned to use to help get across your point, the more grounded you will be in the real world. Your visual aids don't only help the audience understand what you're saying, they are also your allies in keeping you on track.

FOCUS ON RELAXING PHYSICALLY

Take deep breaths, using your diaphragm. Breathe through your nose so you don't get dry mouth. Use simple, unobtrusive isometric techniques. Relax from your feet up: tense different parts of your body and then relax them. To ease neck strain and relax your throat and vocal cords, roll your head in a circle from shoulder to shoulder. Many of these techniques can be used even on stage while you're waiting for your turn to speak.

MAINTAIN EYE CONTACT
WITH THE AUDIENCE

Keep your gaze moving across the audience, but don't look over their heads or at the bridges of their noses. Meet their eyes, one person at a time. You'll be amazed at the open, attentive, interested looks you get back. And if you do meet the eye of someone in the midst of a big yawn, take it in stride, go on, and find someone who's fascinated by what you're saying. Not every single person will be, and it's unrealistic to think otherwise. Keep coming back to the people who are most interested.

"I know it is important to address the audience and talk to them. I seldom stand in one place as I talk but instead I move about with a neck mike. It is good to keep them with you in words and actions. Having given many talks I can usually read the audience. I watch for their facial and body expressions. Are they slumping? Ready to doze? If so I may change the focus or give them a 'red hot' or shocking example to keep their interest. I may ask a question or walk near to them. Most American participants like you to move around, give examples, and use lots of visual aids. Most assuredly, they do not like papers being read to them; it is always best to talk from your paper rather than read it word for word.''

—Madeleine M. Leininger

''Eye contact works though it can be difficult if there are a thousand people there. I try to be expansive in that case, physically turn, gesture to the whole room.''

—William L. Holzemer

''I was invited to give a key note speech. It was the first time I was willing to take on the standard rules of research and provoke thinking in people. My bags got lost en route, including my speech and my slides! I had no reasonable clothes to wear. I spent the night reconstructing the speech as best I could, and gave the speech wearing jeans and Birkenstocks! I must say I got a lot of sympathy for what had happened. People loved it. They were laughing. And it made it easier for me to get across my point that there was another way to think about research. In other words, I used my personal experiences to engage the audience. I had never done this before. I stopped distancing myself from them and tried to share myself, have them know me as I'd want to know them. I confessed the truth to them. Increasingly I use personal stories to lead in. I am more willing to be vulnerable, to show the things I care about.''

—Chris Tanner

Making the Speech

5

WHAT TO DRINK BEFORE YOU SPEAK

- Avoid ice water, which is usually what will be supplied. It constricts your throat just at the moment you want your throat to be open.
- Avoid milk, ice cream, and yogurt. They coat your throat and encourage the production of phlegm.
- Stay away from soda. The carbonation is apt to make you belch.
- Don't drink coffee or tea. The caffeine in both is liable to make you jittery when you need to feel calm.
- No alcohol. You don't want to be *too* calm.
- The best thing to drink for a speaker with a dry throat is cool water with lemon in it. Don't expect this mixture to be available. Bring it with you.
- *Tip of last resort*: Bite your tongue, which causes saliva to flow which moistens your mouth and throat.

LOOK THE AUDIENCE SQUARE IN THE EYE

- Looking directly at people makes them believe you mean what you say. It's also a good way for you to find out if what you're saying is effective.

47

- Look at individuals in the audience, not at the audience in general. Pick out one person and tell her one thing. Pick out another person and tell her the next thing.
- Pretending to look at people, and instead looking at some inanimate object over their heads or to the side, or at the glass of water on their table, fools no one and makes it seem as if there is a reason that you don't want to look at anyone.

> "I try to read faces. Are they nodding, puzzling over things, jotting notes. As opposed to muttering, heads down, with cynical expressions. If this is what's happening, I'll make a joke about it, address it directly. Or I'll change my tactic, use a tried and true story to reengage them. Or I'll interpret back to them what I see in them and ask for their response to this. I'm basically an insecure person and rely on people's feedback and I work hard to get it."
>
> —Chris Tanner

> "The only way to be a successful speaker is to develop a relationship with the audience. I used to be very content oriented. Then I learned that it was more important to relate to them. I chat with the audience. I use humor to get to them. I make Texas jokes. I don't go on to the content until I know they're with me."
>
> —Karlene Kerfoot

THE MICROPHONE

- Don't bend down to meet it. Bring it up to you.
- Don't let it block your face.
- Don't speak while turned away from it.
- Test it to make sure that you don't make "explosions," which happens when you expel too much air into the microphone on certain letter sounds: b, p, s, sh.

YOUR VISUAL AIDS

- Since you've already made sure everyone in the room can see clearly, make sure you don't stand in the way of the projection.

- If the projection is behind you, use a second set of notes so you don't have to turn your head away from the audience.
- Don't move the slides too fast. *You* are familiar with the information on them, but your audience is not, and may want to take notes.

THE POINTER

- Use it sparingly.
- Hold it with the hand closest to the screen.
- Don't wave it around.
- When you're not using it, put it down quietly.
- If you're using a laser pointer, whose beam is invisible and only shows up on the screen as a red dot, be sure you can handle it smoothly. If you can't keep the red dot of light from jumping all over the place, don't use it.

YOUR BODY

- Every gesture carries some meaning. Every posture indicates something about a person—every flick of the wrist, every smile or frown, conveys something to the audience. Therefore, you want to be conscious of what your body is doing, so that it becomes a tool of communication and does not detract from your message.
- You're not an actress, an orator, a sportscaster, a spokesperson, a preacher, a teacher, or a scold. You're a nurse who's giving a talk. So talk to the audience like you would talk to a friend. You know what you want to say, so just say it.
- Don't keep your hands in your pockets or locked behind your back.
- Don't wave your arms or keep your arms crossed.
- Don't jerk your head, nod, shake or use any other habitual gestures that may be distracting.
- Don't drape yourself on the lectern. (*Tip*: Practice at home without it.)

- Don't grip the lectern as if it were a life raft. (*Tip*: Stand to the side of it and concentrate on talking to one person at a time.)

YOUR VOICE

- Breathe deeply to relax and release tension.
- Ask if they can hear you in the back of the room.
- Don't let your pitch creep up into the high register.
- Stop and take a drink if your mouth or throat get dry.

WATCH THE TIME

- Stick to the time you're allotted.
- Keep your watch on the podium, or ask someone in the audience to signal when you have five minutes left to speak.

HECKLERS

If you're speaking and someone who is a problem participant is waving her hand to get your attention, ignore it. It's as simple as that. Don't fixate on her. Since it requires more energy for her to keep waving than for you to keep ignoring her, she'll stop waving before you stop speaking.

If she takes the next step and starts calling out to you, stop speaking for a moment and ask if she'll please hold her question or comment until you're finished. If she keeps shouting, someone from the organization that's invited you to speak, or someone from the hotel or conference center should take care of her. If no one does, ask her once again if she'll hold her questions until you're finished speaking. Whatever you do, don't join the heckler in an argument about freedom of speech or any other topic he/she may want to engage in. Maintain your dignity. If she remains uncooperative, ask for her name. People are usually reluctant to face this challenge, but if this too doesn't shut her up, stop speaking. At this point, you and the audience are both being abused by this person and you must rely on audience support to stop her. If the audience is unable or unwilling to support you, leave.

> "If a person is taking more than their fair turn at the microphone, I would say: 'We all need the opportunity to speak. We've listened to you. Now it's time to move on.'"
>
> —Helen K. Grace

> "If a heckler is asking me questions, I'll use a bridging technique to go from what they're saying to what I'm saying, and then to go on to the next questioner. In other words, I don't always answer the question. Politicians are taught to go into an interview or speech with four points they want to hit and they do that, no matter what the reporter asks them. That's what I do with a heckler or a nay-sayer, someone who says this or that can't work."
>
> —Karlene Kerfoot

QUESTIONS

> "Audiences like to be acknowledged. This is one reason to do question and answer sessions."
>
> —Linda S. Hurwitz

When you plan to have a question-and-answer period after you're done speaking, let your audience know beforehand. You're in control of the question-and-answer period, and you need to set the ground rules before you begin.

- Announce if you'll you take questions during your speech or only afterward.
- Decide if you're going to supply them with blank cards to write their questions.
- Arrange beforehand how these cards will be given out, and then gathered, and then given back to you. This system gives you more control. You can pick and choose which questions

you want to answer. On the other hand, it has less spontaneity and keeps you farther from your audience.

- If audience members are going to ask questions, make sure there is a microphone for them.
- If a questioner cannot be heard by the rest of audience, repeat her question for everyone's benefit.
- Don't feel rushed for an answer. Saying something like: "That is a very interesting question" is a way to give yourself a moment to collect your thoughts before you speak.
- Don't let questions throw you. As a matter of fact, experienced speakers—politicians prominent among them—will tell you that if you don't have an answer to a particular question or if you simply don't want to answer it, acknowledge the question then answer with something you want to say. In other words, use difficult or irrelevant or purposely provocative questions as an opportunity to reinforce your message.
- Announce when there is only time for one question more and only take one question more.

"It is always important to be kind and understanding to the persons asking questions. Never be defensive. Remain open-minded. The audience must feel comfortable and safe to talk with you. Giving keynote addresses is a great honor. It provides wonderful opportunities to share your scholarly ideas with others. But a good keynoter needs to be sensitive to and aware of the audience's needs, responses, and interests. Incorporating the audience's needs into your talk requires a cultural, local knowledge, a lot of listening, thoughtful reflection and rephrasing with examples to be meaningful to the people. I am always interested in their evaluations and request a summary copy. I have always learned from the audience and its cultural variations worldwide. I have been privileged to give nearly 600 addresses, not only to nurses but to other groups and in many places in the world. It has been a wonderful privilege and opportunity to be a transculturally-oriented nurse speaker."

—Madeleine Leininger

"If the questioner is belligerent or angry or disturbed, if they think they know more than you do, if you sense they want the podium, I am always polite. I thank them for their 'interesting' question.

It is never appropriate to embarrass them, though if they're wrong,
I'm not shy about saying so. I always know that, at some point,
the question period will be over and I will be saved by the bell.''

—William L. Holzemer

DON'T BREAK THE SPELL

You've been in charge for the last five or ten or twenty minutes.
You've controlled the atmosphere in the room and you're still in
control. Maintain your posture. Don't slump to show your listeners
how much energy you expended on their behalf. Give the audience
time to let your last words sink in. (In they were good ones, they'll
need that moment to assimilate them and relate them to your
whole speech.)

DON'T APOLOGIZE

Some speakers, so relieved to be done with their speech and to
have gotten through it without a major personal or technical gaffe,
signal their feeling with a big "Phew!" or an expression that says:
"I'm glad that's over!" But it's not over. It's not over until you
graciously accept your audience's applause and go back to your
seat. Even then, save the expression of relief until you're back in
your hotel room. The audience has believed in you, in the sincerity
of your message and in the confident way you gave it; to indicate
that you feel any differently will blunt the lasting effectiveness of
your message and make them lose confidence in you.

THANK THEM FOR THEIR ATTENTION

- Remind the audience that copies of your speech are available.
- Accept the applause with a smile and a nod.

- Make an all-encompassing gesture of good-bye: a wave, a nod of the head, a bow from the waist.

SAY GOOD-BYE

- Spot your exit before you start to move.
- Go directly to it.

Who Owns the Speech?

6

WHOSE SPEECH IS IT, ANYWAY?

OK. You wrote the speech. But does that mean you own it? It is the perception of some organizations that, because they are paying you to make the speech, they also own the rights to it. The surest way to determine who owns the speech you deliver is to discuss it with the sponsoring organization. If you didn't think to do this when the invitation to speak was first extended, make it part of your list of things to discuss with them during your next telephone conversation.

Don't make any assumptions about the organization's policy in this matter. There are many different ways to handle ownership, and you need to know how the particular organization you're dealing with handles it. At one end of the spectrum is the small, young organization, with very little experience in sponsoring speakers. This organization may not have given any thought at all to the matter of who owns the speech. At the other end of the spectrum is the entrenched organization, with a long history of hiring speakers and a policy of ownership firmly in place and ready for your signature on their agreement.

Whatever type of organization you're dealing with, decide your preferences before you speak to them. You may not get exactly what you want; you may have to compromise or accommodate your wants with their needs. In any case, be prepared, so that you are not simply reacting to their policy.

First, don't agree to sign anything up front. If you're pressured to do so during the initial telephone conversation, resist. Say you want to see a copy of the agreement and, once you've read it and considered it, you'll let them know. If the organization has a policy and it's been worked out, reviewed by legal counsel, signed by the president of the organization, and sealed in wax, you still have the right to ask them to send you a copy of the contract or letter of agreement. When you get it, read it carefully. Don't sign it. Read it again.

WHAT IS MEANT BY "RIGHTS OF OWNERSHIP," ANYWAY?

"Owning" a speech means that nothing in the speech can be used without permission. This may mean that people in the audience are not allowed to tape-record the speech while you're giving it, a condition you and the organization who hired you should set in advance. If it's you who doesn't want the speech recorded, be sure to let your audience know, though it sounds less chilly if the person who makes the announcement is the person who introduces you. You may want to prepare a sign that says, "No tape recording permitted during the speech."

The audience may be allowed to take notes, of course, and there really is no way to prevent people from quoting your remarks in a paper they're writing, or a talk they give in the future. If they cite you, which is the polite—not to mention *legal*—thing to do, you ought to be personally and professionally pleased. It certainly does your reputation good to have another nurse give a speech in front of another professional organization and say: "As (your name, properly pronounced, you hope) once said . . . " and then follows it with one of the brilliant remarks you made. The possibility that you might be quoted is a good reason to make sure of the accuracy and relevance of the things you say in your speech. If you say something you wish you hadn't said, or find out later it is incorrect or inaccurate, and then someone quotes you, your reputation suffers.

KNOW WHAT YOU WANT THE FUTURE OF YOUR SPEECH TO BE

If the organization requested that you give them a paper as well as make a speech, and you have agreed to do this, the organization may assume that you have also given them the right to publish it. That doesn't sound so bad, you may say to yourself. After all, publication means that your audience is not only the people in the auditorium who actually hear you, but also all those people out there who will read your speech in its published form. And the more people you reach with your ideas, the better. All this is true, of course. Nevertheless, don't let your eagerness to increase your audience go against a more prudent, and ultimately wiser, course of action. There are several things you ought to consider before you agree to this offer.

You may want to retain the rights to the speech so you can use it again. That speech that you're so eager to disseminate to the mass reading audience may, in fact, be the speech that will see you through a hundred speaking engagements over the next few years. It may be the speech that gets you a job offer, or offers to speak in front of other groups, or interviewed by the press. It may be the speech that will make you famous. Of course, you'll have to update certain facts, use the most current statistics, and change the names of a few politicians here and there to keep it up to date. But it is a good speech, isn't it? It was good enough to get you the offer of publication from the organization, wasn't it? Remember that, if it is published by this organization, all that juicy information, all those terrific jokes, brilliant insights, dazzling statistics, and startling conclusions that you worked so hard to research and polish, have just been co-opted. And the person who has done the co-opting is none other than yourself. Remember that you can't give it away and still have it too.

You may also want to find out how the organization intends to publish your speech. Their publication procedure may not be to your liking. You cannot assume that an organization's publishing capability is on par with the size and importance of the organization itself. You may be very mistaken about this. A professional nursing organization, no matter how large, is not a publishing company. Their ability to publish your speech may be woefully inadequate. Their journal or newsletter distribution may be quite limited. Their production facilities may display the speech in a way that is less than ideal. You may imagine a privately printed reprint in four colors; they may run off a hundred black-and-white copies on a photocopying machine. Their lack of experience or personnel for the task may severely limit the amount of publicity your speech will get if published in this fashion. Ads in nursing journals cost money. Direct mailings to advertise the publication also cost. Does the organization have the money and expertise to assume distribution? Find out.

You also ought to know the context in which your speech will be published. Will it stand alone? Will it be included as part of a series of papers? Who are the other authors? If some of the top nursing speakers in the country are going to be included, you may want to see your speech in this good company.

Finally, you may not want your speech or paper published in a proceedings when, with a little expert editorial work (more on this in Chapter 7), you might be able to sell it to a nursing journal. This could result in a much wider readership, in addition to professional level editing, polishing, publicity, and wide distribution. Or, you may acknowledge all of these things and still agree to let the organization publish your paper, while stipulating that you will retain the rights to submit it for republication after theirs is out. Whatever you decide to do, find out all the information and decide what to do before you give the speech.

THE ORGANIZATION'S RIGHT
TO RECORD THE SPEECH

Again, going in, you must decide if you will permit them to tape-record you. If you do, are you giving the organization the rights to sell that tape recording of your speech? If you do grant them the right, do you want a percentage of the profits from the sale? The organization may perceive that, since they have paid you to make the speech, they own it. If this is not discussed up front, problems could ensue. You might feel that you have been badly used and that they are making profits on your work. On the other hand, if you go on and get the work published, they may feel you are cutting in on their sales.

If you are going to go along with the taping, and know the organization is going to sell the tape, find out how much the tape is going to sell for and about how many people it is likely to reach. It may be very flattering to be asked to have your speech taped and merchandised, and even profitable. On the other hand, if you were planning to give this speech again and again in the future, you may not want it taped and reused. If people have the tape, they may not need you.

GIVE CREDIT WHERE CREDIT IS DUE

If you are quoting from someone in your speech, you must cite them with as much care and respect and attention to what is legal and right as you would when citing them in a written paper for a nursing journal. This applies whether you are quoting them exactly, paraphrasing their idea, or taking off from an idea of theirs as a starting point.

Although, in principle, a citation is a citation, in practice they are different. In a paper you would number the quote and write a complete reference that would include the author's name, the name of the book or journal in which the quote appeared originally, the page number, where and when it was printed, the publisher, and date. When someone is reading an article, there is plenty of time for them to make a note of the citation when they finish reading the whole article. In a speech, you need to keep the audience's attention, so a long citation would obviously be inappropriate. The last thing you want to do is bore your audience. All you need to do is say, "As so and so once said, 'A good idea is one that isn't overly familiar or too strange.'" Using quotes is a little like being judged by the company you keep, so choose your quotes carefully.

If your speech is filled with quotes from lots of different people, all you need to do is mention their names and tell the audience that you'll pass out a bibliography later. This will relieve the audience from feeling they have to spend all the time you're speaking writing down the names of the people you're quoting. Instead, you want them listening to you. By the way, the bibliography should conform to the way you write one for an article.

Using quotes without giving credit to the person you're quoting, or using someone's ideas without mentioning that you've done so, is the verbal equivalent of plagiarism. Verbal plagiarism won't get you in the kind of trouble that literary plagiarism will, but, if you're found out, it will do something just as bad: destroy your credibility. People will think: if she used that quote and didn't cite the person, how do we know that she hasn't done the same with all her other brilliant ideas? Once that kind of doubt sets in, either during the speech or afterward, listeners will have difficulty trusting you again.

WHAT COULD HAPPEN WHEN YOU DON'T PROTECT YOURSELF?

One prominent nurse, the author of many books, tells a story that should curl anyone's hair. She had given a series of lectures based on a book she was in the process of writing. One of her most gifted nursing students took copious notes during all the lectures and, a year and a half later, came out with a book whose contents were derived totally from these lecture notes.

Transforming a Speech into a Paper; A Paper into a Speech

7

SCENARIO #1:

You've just given a successful speech: the audience is attentive, the question-and-answer period lively, compliments as to content and delivery rain upon you. Afterward you are approached by the editor of a professional nursing journal, who happens to be in the audience. Your speech, she says, would be a wonderful addition to her journal and could you just rewrite it as an article. Flattered, you say yes, and set about the simple task of typing up the speech and mailing it off.

Not so fast.

On the one hand, it does seem like a simple and natural thing to do. You've done all the research needed to give a successful speech and organized the material in a thoughtful, coherent way, so why not simply turn it into a paper, have it published, and increase the size of your audience?

SCENARIO #2:

You've written a terrific article that's been published in a prestigious journal. A few months later, you get a call from a professional nursing organization, asking you to speak on the same topic you covered so thoroughly in your article. Flattered—and thinking there is so little to do to convert the material—you agree. In fact, you think, it may be possible simply to read the article out loud as it is, without changing a word. After all, you worked hard on the material. There's no reason not to capitalize on the work you've done by creating two exposures for a single effort.

Slow down.

Sometimes this transition from one medium to the other actually succeeds and, theoretically, there is no reason why you shouldn't try to make one serve the other. But there are several significant differences between a speech that is written to be spoken aloud and a paper that is written to be read silently. There are more than a few pitfalls to watch out for when making the conversion.

SIMILARITIES BETWEEN A SPEECH AND A PAPER

Audience Attention

In both forms you have to get the attention of your audience— reader or listener—right from the start, or they won't be there when you finish. If it's a speech and you've failed to do so, you'll feel their lack of interest as it's translated into coughing, fidgeting, stifled yawning, the sounds of cellophane rattling as they unwrap hard candy; the sight of sleeves pushed gently back to check their watches. If it's a paper, mercifully, you won't see a thing, but you can imagine the sound of the journal closing and being tossed on the pile of other journals either already read or destined to go unread.

Organization

In both a speech and a paper, the organizational rule remains the same: Tell them what you're going to tell them (the Introduction); tell them (the Body of the speech or paper); tell them what you just told them (the Closing).

WHAT'S APPROPRIATE IN A SPEECH MAY NOT WORK IN A PAPER

Visuals

Although visuals are an important part of any speech, their impact can be felt even more powerfully when you convert the speech to a paper. (Conversely, you should be aware that the graph that works so well on the page, will lose some of its impact when you make it part of your speech. Size alone accounts for much of this.)

In a speech, you will have the advantage of different visual forms: video, film, slides, and a laser pointer, posters, charts, and music. Most of these won't translate at all to the page and the ones that do—charts and posters—will be reduced in size and impact. On the other hand, graphic details do not work very well during a speech, but stand a good chance of being studied when the reader can hold it in her hand and peruse it at her own speed.

Questions

In a speech, you may ask a question of the audience and actually get an answer. The answer may stimulate other questions, which may invoke answers you didn't know you knew. Knowledge may increase exponentially and this can be both lively and stimulating. In a paper, a question may serve to stimulate further thought on the part of the reader, but it is rhetorical, in that you expect no answer; you are prodding the reader to think about an answer and then, because you cannot know for certain what their answer will be, you must go on without the answer. In an article, there is no give-and-take between writer and reader, as there may well be between speaker and audience.

Personal Information

Personalizing information is often a way to bridge the information gap between you and your audience. Whether this takes the form of an anecdote, a funny story, or the relating of an incident that occurred on your way to the speaking engagement, it works by creating a bond between speaker and audience, helped by the speaker's personality. As a technique it is usually too informal to make the successful transition to a written paper.

Timeliness

A speech can take advantage of the fact that it can be rewritten, added to, subtracted from, amended, appended, and altered in just about any way you can think of, in order to take advantage of the current state of the world. Let's say a nurse is scheduled to give a paper on the latest trends in home care. The day before she is scheduled to give her talk, the state legislature passes a new bill that alters home care reimbursement. No problem; with not much effort, she can work that event into her speech.

Turning that speech into a paper has to take into account the fact that today's news is tomorrow's history. Because there is such a long lead time—often as long as a full year—between the day an article has been accepted for publication and the day that article appears in print, timeliness can never be one of the strong points of a written article.

Form

A speech is most effective when it is linear, that is, when it states its theme and objective, and follows it in a clear path to its conclusion. Any digression, any branching off into illustrative examples, assumes that the audience is keeping track of the main point and will have no difficulty following the speaker back to it when the digression is complete. This is a lot to assume of a listening audience, no matter how willing and cooperative they might be.

An article, however, may use many branching ideas with the confidence that the reader can refer back to the main point if she gets lost—and if the main point is sufficiently compelling to warrant this extra work. A carefully planned article allows for structured digression.

Accuracy of Information

Although this may be considered controversial by some editors, an article need only be accurate and informative in order to accomplish its basic purpose. If the information is something the reader wants to get, she will plow through even the dullest article to get it. A speech must also be accurate and informative; in addition, it must be entertaining, for the simple reason that someone listening to a dull speech, no matter how well intentioned that listener might be, will have to exercise superhuman effort to remain alert if the speech is dull.

References

An article may take advantage of the very nature of the way people learn, by providing extensive references, citations, bibliography, charts, and examples; in short, by being comprehensive and complex. The reader of an article can go back and reread a portion of the article, hold up a chart next to another chart, or take notes in the margin for later reference. The listener to a speech can do none of these things, so, in adapting an article to a speech, the writer must simplify, choose the references that are most important, as well as choose the charts and the examples for maximum impact.

WHAT DOESN'T TRANSLATE FROM THE STAGE TO THE PAGE?

The flesh impact of a spoken speech is completely lost in a written article. The very power of your personality, the force of your delivery, the impression your physical self makes in gesture, body language, and vocal inflections is not present when you convert the speech to a paper. As a result, you must be very certain, when making this conversion, that language itself is an adequate substitute.

In fact, all the trappings of an in-person speech will not be at your disposal if you convert your speech into a paper. You will not be able to welcome the audience, assess them by age or gender, praise them, make eye contact with them, guide them, respond to them, question them, or answer their questions, much less thank them for their attention.

DIFFERENT WAYS PEOPLE TAKE IN INFORMATION

There are many ways in which the attention a reader brings to an article is more reliable than that which she brings to a lecture or speech. The people in an audience are subject to many influences not under their control: the size and temperature of the room, the comfort of their chair, their view of the speaker, and the speed at which the speaker speaks. Their choice of clothing is apt to be formal.

Are they there because they have chosen to be there willingly? Are they interested in the subject, or has their Nurse Manager required them to attend? Are they away for the weekend at a resort and eager to get out and take a swim? Whether or not the people in the audience know each other plays a large part in how well they listen. If they know a lot of the people in the audience and, hence, feel the pressure of retaining the content of the speech, they are apt to pay better attention than if they are in a room full of strangers, to whom they owe nothing.

A reader of a paper, on the other hand, is reading it for only one of two reasons: she is required to read it for a course she is taking or to keep up on her field of interest or expertise; or she is simply interested in the subject. A reader is in control of the time she is giving to reading and the environment in which she is doing it. She has chosen the chair, the lighting, the room temperature, and the clothes she is wearing. Most importantly, she may take in the information at her own speed, going over what she didn't get the first time, savoring passages, making notes, underlining.

DIFFERENCES BETWEEN A LISTENING AND A READING VOCABULARY

People have four different vocabularies: the largest vocabulary is the reading one; people recognize words as they read whose precise—or even general—meaning they may not actually know or be able to define, apart from context. Related to this is the writing vocabulary, those words each person has available with which to express thoughts; this may often be augmented by the use of dictionaries and other reference materials and by rewriting and editing. The third vocabulary is the listening one; people are able to understand words spoken aloud, often helped by the speaker's gesture, inflection, and body language, in addition to context. The fourth, and smallest vocabulary, are those words available to our own extemporaneous speech: the words we have at our disposal in daily conversation.

In order to convert a paper to a speech or a speech to a paper most successfully, it is necessary to understand that there is a basic difference in the ways people comprehend language. Simply put: language that is to be comprehended through listening ought to be simpler and bolder than language that is to be comprehended through reading.

WHY MAKE THE CONVERSION AT ALL?

Money?

No matter how high your hopes or diligent your work, know from the outset that rare is the nurse who got rich writing articles for professional journals or giving speeches in front of professional nursing organizations. Converting a speech to a paper or vice versa is not likely to make you any richer than sticking with the original form. There are compelling reasons, however, to make the conversion.

Reaching a Wider Audience

If you've given a speech, the audience is likely to range from 25 people to a few hundred; even if you've given the same speech a dozen times, the audience is relatively small when considered in the context of the amount of nurses there are who you believe ought to get the information you're presenting. A speech is evanescent. Once you've given it, it exists only in the memories of the people who heard it; its main impact came at the time you gave it and declines thereafter, except as it may have influenced, by the persuasive aspects of the spoken word, the actions of the people who heard it. Converting the speech into an article increases your audience by introducing the material to the readership of the journal in which the article appears. To be published as an article gives the information a longer life; the journal will remain in people's personal collections, on library shelves, on microfilm, in computer data banks, available to research for . . . dare it be said? . . . *forever.*

Reaching a Smaller Audience

If size is so important, why ever would you want to convert an article into a speech and reach only a hundred people when the article has already reached a thousand? Because there is nothing quite so satisfying as walking into a room of people and, just by the force of your ideas and personality, convincing them of your point of view, educating them, making converts, goading them into action, making them question their assumptions. Something like this may happen when they read your article, but you will not be there to see it, nor will the way you give the speech help to put those ideas across.

Personal Satisfaction

In addition to the satisfaction of increasing your audience or getting more personal with it, there is something private to be gained in the very act of conversion: an intellectual game played by yourself in which you are forced to rethink your subject from a slightly different angle. The results—in clarity and new insights—can often be very rewarding.

Other Forms
of Oral Communication

8

Speech making is only one form of oral communication. In the ordinary course of an ordinary day, most nurses will be involved in other forms: staff meetings, interviews, panel discussions, group discussions, one-on-one conversations, and telephone conversations. The same principles that apply to more formal public speaking also apply to these less formal arenas. The ability to make oneself understood, to communicate clearly, efficiently, and persuasively, is a necessary part of every nurse's personal and professional equipment.

PANEL DISCUSSIONS

These often follow a speech and so the members should be chosen for their relevance to the speaker's subject matter. For small groups, there is no more congenial setting than the round table. For gatherings of forty or more, the appropriate setting of the panel forum is an arc or V seating pattern, since this enables the group of panelists to see each other and to be seen by an audience. There's nothing less conducive to lively discussion than panelists seated next to each other in a row, who then have to crane their necks to see who's speaking.

There is a limited number of people who can appear on a panel and still have them all be effective, so keep the number between three and ten. This is large enough to include a variety of opinions on a shared subject, yet small enough for informal interchange among them and, later, with those out front.

Creating the Panel

When you're on a program committee, planning an event, one of your responsibilities is the organization of the panel. Before personnel choices come up for discussion, you and your co-committee members must choose the topic. Once your topic is firmly in place, it's the job of the committee to discuss, search for, and select the people who will sit on the panel. There are certain qualities these people ought to have and certain questions you should ask of yourself in order to determine the person's appropriateness: How well can the person you're considering represent a particular point of view on the topic? How expert are they in the field? How well are they likely to handle themselves in a panel discussion?

The people you consider don't have to be famous in their field, but if they are, it is wise to approach them well in advance of the actual panel, since these people are often booked a long time ahead.

When trying to select the people to make up a panel, there are three primary roles to consider, each requiring different skills and personal qualities. In your career as a nurse, you may be sitting on the committees to select people to play these roles, or you may be called upon to play any one of them yourself.

The Moderator

The qualities you need to fulfill this role are often a combination of opposites. You need to be calm and cool, but also firm. You need to speak distinctly and clearly, though not formally, since you won't be giving a speech. You need to be patient with everyone, while, at the same time, keeping to a time schedule. You need to be generous and sympathetic to all who speak, and also confident enough to be able to stop people from rambling. You need to be modest enough to sit back and let the discussion proceed at its own pace, with its own twists and turns, but commanding enough of people and the topic itself to guide discussion if it goes astray.

Once you've accepted the role of moderator and the event has begun, you'll introduce each person on the panel, giving their essential credits. The committee should have decided beforehand on an arbitrary number of lines for this introduction, so that everyone is treated equally and, if they haven't, it is up to you to even things out. You don't want the discussion to be prematurely weighted in favor of the panelist with the longest list of accomplishments, or handicap someone else with a short list. (If someone's accomplishments are dauntingly lengthy, just hit the high spots.) At the end of the introductions, you'll make a statement as to how the proceedings will be carried out, saying, for example, that each panel member will speak for five minutes. The committee will have informed you and the panelists of this time limit well in advance, but it is up to you to reiterate it and see that they adhere to it.

A panel is not a series of small speeches. The committee may have instructed the members to begin with a short introduction of their position. After these introductory remarks are made, you must see to it that the majority of panel time is spent in active exchange among the panelists. (It's up to you to cut short—politely—an inconsiderate panel member who tries to turn her time for introductory remarks into a full-blown speech. The committee and the audience expect and rely on you to exercise this kind of control.)

For the most part, you should keep yourself out of the panel discussion, except to move it along. The committee has probably structured the event so that a reasonable amount of the time (a quarter to a third) is reserved for questions from the listeners. It is up to you to make this clear when the introductions have been concluded. If the audience is shy or reluctant to speak, it is up to you to encourage them. Since you have been chosen partly because you know the listeners and their areas of expertise, you might call on a particular person with expert knowledge and ask them to add to what has been said by the panel. You might also turn to the panel itself for expansion or clarification of some statements that had been made. It is also up to you to see that every panelist gets a chance to speak. If necessary, you may need to step in with a direct request: "I'd like to know what you think on that point, Ms. Carter . . . " And, of course, you can turn to members of the committee or even ask questions of the panel members yourself.

When the allotted time has been filled, it's your job to sum things up. This requires you to bring together the various paths followed in the discussion. You'll need to take notes during the discussion to prepare for this summation. (You ought to make sure to have an adequate supply of writing equipment available.) Your goal is for the listeners to leave the discussion with a clear synthesis of the main ideas, and the panelists to feel they have been well and fairly served by the summation.

You should draw the meeting to a close, while the attention of the listeners is still enthusiastic. The panelists and the audience should be thanked and, as the applause for all dies down, the meeting ends on a high note.

The Panelist

If you've been asked to sit on a panel, there's probably a good reason for the invitation. You're recognized as someone whose opinions on the topic are worth hearing. You would not have been asked to join as a panel member if this were not the case. Don't let modesty stand in the way of agreeing to participate. The gains are many: an increase in confidence, positive feedback, and a public forum to communicate your ideas.

Your preparation will be modest, since you have been asked to be on a panel to discuss a subject in which you are already well versed. However, you may want to jot down a few notes about things you want to be sure to say. You will not be giving a speech, but you want to be sure that your most significant points are made clearly. Beyond that, your preparation has been going on for years. (You may also want to refer back in this volume for the rules governing any discussion, so you'll know what to expect in terms of the forum in which you'll be speaking. Don't assume that those inviting you to be on a panel will use this format accurately. Ask if you're expected to give a short speech before the discussion. Ask for the time anticipated, if this is the case.)

Once you are on the panel, there are a few things to keep in mind. You and the other panel members are participating in a cooperative enterprise. Though panel members may disagree on things, this is not a debate. No one is trying to "win" anything, but simply to air their views. In order for the event to run smoothly, you'll want to treat the moderator in a supportive manner. You'll also want to adhere to the rules the moderator has set forth. If you have five minutes to make a statement, don't take longer. If you do and the moderator is doing her job, you will be cut off before you have time to finish.

If you and another panel member or an audience member find yourselves in disagreement, attack the point, not the person ("I disagree with what you're saying" instead of : "You don't know what you're talking about."). Don't raise your voice in argument. Spend your energy instead in trying to make your point as clearly as you can. Concentrate on putting forth a convincing case. One of the ways to do this is to listen to the other members of the panel as carefully as you hope they are listening to you. In this way, the discussion may reach heights of logic and truth finding that would be impossible if the participants were arguing to win.

The Listener

Not being the moderator and not on the panel does not exempt you from active participation in the discussion. Listening, in fact, is often harder than speaking, because the act of speech itself keeps the speaker grounded and concentrating. If you regard listening as passive, you're likely to drift off and stop listening.

Paying attention means giving energy to those in front of you. Before the panel has even begun, you as a listener should be thinking about the subject at hand. This way you'll know what issues might be raised and already have some opinions about them. Take notes while the panelists are speaking. Jot down things you want to ask questions about, things you agree with wholeheartedly and want to pledge your support to, or things you totally disagree with and believe need further clarification. When question times comes, don't shrink back and let shyness dominate your curiosity. Group spirit of cooperation and communication should be the thing that drives you to raise the points you thought of, while the panelists were speaking. In this context, shyness may be no different than selfishness. Concentrate instead on the purpose of your question: to communicate and activate others to communicate.

When the audience asks questions, the outcome of the entire panel discussion is increased exponentially in terms of the vitality of the participation and the reality of the goals reached. As an active, listening member of the event, it is up to you to give back to the people who have given to you.

DISCUSSION GROUPS

In the normal course of events, though fewer nurses will actually face a large audience, many will participate regularly in business conferences, staff meetings, caucuses, union and executive board meetings, and committee meetings. They'll also participate in study groups, research teams, and fund-raising collectives.

These groups have many obvious differences, often in terms of content. They also have much in common based on their structure. All of these group meetings pose challenges rooted in group dynamics and solutions grounded in conversation. They promise positive payoffs when approached and attended to with improved oral communication skills. Those of you who do well in these groups—and cause the groups themselves to succeed—are those of you who can promote fluency and self-expression.

In a discussion group, people discuss things, meaning, according to the *Random House Dictionary*, "to consider or examine by argument, comment, etc. Especially to explore solutions. Synonyms: debate, deliberate, reason."

Leading a Group

"Some people are natural leaders, and some people aren't, and there's nothing anybody can do about that."

Like many false assumptions, this one is based on the fact that some people have learned how to recognize, develop, and use the skills they have, in order to take a leadership position, while others have let shyness, reluctance, and/or laziness reinforce their feelings of inadequacy. While the "natural" leader seems to come to the role as if born to it, in fact, she has realized early on that the skills for leadership are quantifiable and therefore learnable, and she has put herself to the test and learned how to lead.

These nurses will tell you that leadership is not magical. It does not involve "getting people to do what you want them to do." It *does* involve the willingness to deal with problems, to assume responsibility for outcomes, to know how to listen to others, to use their knowledge and experience, and to credit them for it. No leader leads alone.

When you assume a leadership position, a magic aura will not surround you. Your personality will not change, though you may feel more confident and powerful just by virtue of having assumed the role. You will not automatically know what to do, just as people will not automatically give you a leader's power just because of your position. There are simply a series of tasks to be faced and goals to be accomplished, and a straight road to take to get where you want to go. When you accept or volunteer to chair a committee, moderate a panel, or lead a group discussion, you have given yourself an opportunity to learn how to function as a leader. Here are some of the things you will need to do:

- Understand the problems facing the group.
- Know the group's goals.
- Make a list of things that need to be discussed.
- Check the accuracy of this list before the meeting, and ask for changes and suggestions.
- Set up a protocol for how group members will indicate a desire to speak.
- Listen very carefully to everyone.
- Keep the discussion on the issues, not on personalities, especially when conflicts arise.
- Ask questions that relate to the topic.
- Restate the topic and the goals when the discussion begins to stray.
- Don't judge the speakers, but do keep things on track in terms of what is germane to the topic.

- If the discussion is becoming mired in irrelevancies or details, help people unstick themselves.

LEADERSHIP PROBLEMS

Some leaders are not the leaders they think they are. Watch that you don't become one of these.

Not Enough of a Leader

She's too democratic. In her desire to be democratic, she winds up not exercising any guidance. She's apt to come to a meeting without a prepared agenda, in the belief that she should not force her ideas on the group. She doesn't lead the discussion, because she doesn't want to impede the free flow of ideas. She doesn't call people to account because she wants to avoid seeming dictatorial. The result of this supposedly democratic position is anarchy.

Too Much of a Leader

At the opposite pole is the leader who believes it is up to her to know both the problem and the solution, too. Admittedly, there are nurses who do this and succeed at it. Of course, she gets all the credit when her solution works. On the other hand, when her solution fails, she is apt to point to the group itself and suggest that, if only they had cooperated with her, her plan would not have failed.

QUESTIONS AND ANSWERS

As the leader, one of your responsibilities is to handle the questions and answers from those present, whether they are an audience for a speech or panel discussion, or other members of a discussion group. Here is what you need to do when taking questions:

- Make sure that everyone in the room and in the audience can hear the question. If people haven't heard it, repeat it yourself, using volume that you know reaches everyone.

- If a question is vague, ask for clarification or reword it, so that it makes the questioner's point more succinctly.
- Encourage questions as a way of sharing information, even if you have to point out particular people whose expertise you know.
- Politely disregard questions that are off the topic.

FUNCTIONING IN A GROUP

When you and others gather at a conference, a panel discussion, or a group meeting, a cooperative effort should be made to put forth ideas in an atmosphere of mutual respect and regard, and to work toward mutual solutions of a problem. Most of us have been in group discussions in which none of this happens. It is clear that the mere getting together of a group of people is no guarantee that respect will be present, and that solutions will either be worked toward or arrived at. The reason for the lack of success of many groups is the lack of agreed-upon rules. Following are some you can all say yes to up front and work with successfully.

Focus on the Problem, Not on the Solution

It's natural to want to make progress in a meeting, and finding a solution is often the surest sign that progress has been made. But, in reality, if the first thing you and your group do is jump to a conclusion, you'll probably have to rethink the problem. It may seem that "brainstorming" or "kicking around ideas" in a group is time-consuming and wasteful, and is not really work. But, by not jumping to a conclusion but instead considering the problem carefully, time is saved and the whole process usually turns out to be productive. So, before you and your group start throwing solutions on the table . . .

Communicate, Communicate, Communicate, Communicate, Communicate

It can't be said too many times. Keep in mind that, unless you make yourself clearly understood, you have no chance of convincing anyone of your point of view. First of all, you have to be heard to be convincing, so speak up, clearly and distinctly. Don't avoid going to meetings because you're not sure you've got all your communication skills down pat. Challenge yourself. Learn by doing. Ask for feedback from people you trust. Your experiences in group communication will teach you more than you could teach yourself by practicing at home alone or complaining about how others hog all the time.

Continue to brush up your skills in voice, vocabulary, and conversation. Remember how large a role is played by body language. You may even want to try out a role-playing group with some friends before your actual meeting. Once you're able to convince your friends of something, the people at the meeting will be easier (though not necessarily easy) to handle. Listen carefully to whomever is speaking.

Open Your Mind and Keep It Open

We all know what it's like to have our own point of view so clearly in mind that we don't even hear what other people are saying. All we are doing is waiting until that other person is finished speaking so we can say what we have to say. This is a description of a mind that is closed to new ideas.

In a group, what should be kept in mind is the common goal. To this end, we should all train ourselves to listen to and sincerely try to understand the views and beliefs of others. No one gains if we all believe we're right and everyone else is wrong. Don't waste time vindicating your mistakes and vilifying the suggestions of others. Remember, in the Middle Ages, one of the seven deadly sins was self-justification.

Listen Efficiently, Test Your Recall, Stop Smiling

We've all experienced it: someone is talking in a group and we realize we are nodding and smiling and exhibiting all the signs of the attentive listener, when, in fact, our minds are a million miles away and we haven't heard a thing the speaker has said. This charade gets no one anywhere—not you, not the person speaking, and certainly not the group.

We should all strive to remember things when we hear them. One way to test ourselves is by restating in our own words what's just been said. The result of ineffective listening is that the group's ability to act and react is crippled. When this happens, it is the end of group discussion, no matter how many people are smiling.

Obey the Informal Dictates of the Group

Discussion groups are generally informal. A scheme of behavior as codified in *Roberts' Rules of Order* is not necessarily applicable, or even helpful. There are, however, procedures that we should all agree upon. As with panel discussions, there is a leader who guides the discussion, rather than dictates, and keeps the meeting on track without taking over.

There is a back-and-forth, give-and-take relationship between members. People are encouraged—by the leader and by the group members themselves—to speak and to contribute their ideas. Interpersonal relationships are fostered by the group. All of this should happen in an atmosphere that is relaxed and free of the formal constraints imposed by rigid rules of procedure. It is up to the leader to keep the group from getting mired in such procedures and thereby obscuring the issues.

Come to a Group Meeting Prepared

If you as a group member are not well prepared, you are doing a disservice to the group, because poorly informed members are bound to reach poorly informed decisions. If you've all convened to make a decision, see if you can avoid wasting a lot of time deciding that you're going to make a decision. Skip that stalling step and get right to it.

Prepare any way you like. Go over your thoughts the night before the meeting, or even on your way to work. Take a ten-minute break before the meeting, and walk around the block. Use this time to organize your ideas. Jot down a few notes and refer to any other notes you've made. Just be sure that, whatever your preparation is, it's enough for you to take an active and significant part in the discussion.

Argue with Issues, Not with People

Observe those people in the group who take out their own feelings of anger and frustration on other individuals or on the group as a whole. When you find yourself having those feelings, try to see the people with whom you disagree as the co-workers and group members they are, people whose trust and empathy is important to you. It is certainly a fact of life that not everyone is going to have an opinion that you agree with, but, in terms of group discussion, everyone's opinion is worthy of your respectful attention.

Those individuals who like to argue often do so by targeting weak spots in others. In a real give-and-take discussion, the aim is to get past our own opinions and look to the larger picture painted by the group as a whole. To do this, we need to free ourselves from the temptation to label and categorize everyone present and resist the urge to attack a person, when what we are really disagreeing with is that person's opinion. Maintenance of group harmony should be part of every group member's goal.

Maintain Individuality

Caving in on particular personal beliefs when faced with the growing pressure of majority opinion is an ever-present trap in group discussion. Oftentimes, you may not feel secure enough in your opinions to oppose the group, and so you'll wait until the meeting is over and then regale your trusted friends with your true feelings. It is your responsibility, the responsibility of each member of the group, and of the group as a whole to hear out all minority opinions, even those of the group's shyest members.

You should never allow a majority to intimidate you into silence. Such shyness is often a mask of superiority toward the group, as if you're saying, "I know better, but I'm not going to take the trouble of telling anyone." Stand up for your opinions and beliefs, no matter what the group says or thinks. Great ideas often stem from minority opinions.

Avoid Traditional Thinking

We often find comfort in the tried and true, but those ways of thinking often stand in the way of creative solutions to problems.

No one ever rode a train to the future while standing still at the station. Freedom of thought can't thrive when you want to preserve the status quo. Progress can't be made when you feel the need to snuggle in with the comfortable old ways of doing things. This is not to suggest we throw out everything we know, but instead to recognize that it takes effort and courage to look for new ways to see old problems.

You and the group should not hesitate to make a clean break with the traditional ways of doing things, at least in the discussion stages. No idea should be rejected just because it has never been brought up before. Nor should any idea be clung to just because it has worked in the past.

Ask Probing Questions

In group discussion, questions can often be more important than answers—more challenging, more thought provoking—and should be posed with that in mind. They should not be asked rhetorically. They should not answer themselves. They should not be veiled threats, meant to stifle potential answers. Questions should be asked in such a way as to encourage responsive answers and to help move the discussion along productive lines.

Appropriate questions are those concerning statements or facts that can be verified; those of interpretation; those of value, in which assessments are made of comparative merit and questions of policy, those which define aims and goals. These kinds of questions are a solid grounding for reasoned, persuasive group discussion. As the group searches for answers to its own problems, probing questions can be used to uncover the weaknesses in arguments and the fallacies in ways of thinking.

Be Sensitive to the Intricacies of Language

A word may mean one thing to you and an entirely different thing to the person sitting next to you. Misunderstandings like this arise from the different experiences people have had with language. When speaking to a group of people, it is easy to be misunderstood by the casual use of a word that suggests several meanings.

Be mindful of those words or expressions that stop the flow of information and rational discourse. These include idioms, regional slang, labels affixed to any group, clichés that cloak themselves as experience, insider language that outsiders find incomprehensible, shorthand talk that encourages shorthand thinking, ambiguity and vagueness, especially those inherent in such empty expressions as "you know" and "et cetera." If you've got this verbal cotton candy in your speech, become aware of it and try to eliminate it. Ask yourself what you really mean, and then say what you really mean. If someone else is using this idiomatic language, ask her to explain herself more clearly.

> "A nurse manager can't succeed without being able to speak well in public. You want to ascend the nursing ladder because you have something to sell: yourself, the way you lead, your beliefs. If you're not going to change people's behavior, you can't lead. If you're not a good public speaker, you can't sell things or influence people. Even if the speaking is just to a group of two or three, the same principles apply. You have to make it fun to be in the group. If the group isn't with you, the work doesn't get done. It's good to think of the group as people who are evaluating you, then try harder."
>
> —Karlene Kerfoot

INTERVIEWS

At some point in your career as a nurse you are going to be called upon to conduct any number of different kinds of interviews or participate as the person being interviewed, sometimes in your search for a new job, sometimes to ask for a raise, to seek a promotion or change of duties, to answer questions about work-related problems, perhaps on television or radio or by the print media.

When you are doing the interviewing—be it to hire someone, to find out information from a staff member or colleague, from someone friendly, neutral, or hostile—you are in charge and there are ways to get what you want.

When you are being interviewed, there are ways to say what you want to say without being manipulated into saying what you had no intention of saying. The skills any nurse needs to go into these interviews and come out of them successfully are the same skills that are required in all forms of successful speech:

- Ideas must be clearly thought through and well organized.
- The person doing the interviewing must be analyzed, which means careful listening.
- A goal must be kept in mind from which you do not stray.

Preparation Is the Key

In this respect, the interview is similar to all other forms of public speaking. If you are clear when you go into an interview as to what you want to achieve, you will be able to maximize your ability to handle anything unplanned or unexpected that might arise. In fact, it is just as important to chart the course of your interview as it is to get yourself ready to write and deliver a formal speech. In other respects, the interview is different, because the interviewer has major control over the direction of the conversation.

Ask yourself this question: "What am I trying to achieve with this interview?" It doesn't matter whether you have requested the interview yourself or have been summoned to it by a superior. When the interview is with the media, setting a clear objective is even more important.

With the question in mind, construct an outline of how the interview ideally should go. Determine the purpose you want to achieve—the direction you want the conversation to take. Don't be surprised if the actual interview veers away from what you have planned; chances are more likely than not that it will. But the outline you've created and put to memory will serve you well as a series of reference points. Knowing what you want to say and the shape of the interview as a whole will give you a structure to which you can return. This structure will help you stay on track and also give you the confidence to go with the flow of the interview.

Formal Interview

In a formal interview the questions are to the point, and so your answers should be simple and clear. If the question is general ("What did you do in school?") you need to be able to distinguish between a trivial answer ("I was on the tennis team.") and an important one ("I worked on my Masters in Oncological Nursing."). By focusing on what is truly important, you'll also curb the tendency to chit-chat, which happens to people when they are in a tension-producing situation.

Informal Interview

The informal interview often feels like a free-form friendly talk in a relaxed style that seems to have no structure at all. It is often more effective in eliciting information than the more rigid question-and-answer format. Its apparent ease allows you to let down those formal barriers and actually have a conversation, in which you are encouraged to speak your mind more openly. The person doing the interview now has the advantage of getting not only information from you, but a more instinctive sense of who you are, your character, and your personality.

But, don't be fooled by the informality of this type of interview; it is still an interview and, though the conversation may seem to be casual and without an apparent agenda, skilled interviewers will be pursuing their goals nevertheless. It's up to you to remember to accomplish your own. The key to this kind of interview is to listen. If you do so carefully—not just to the question or remark, but to the purpose that underlies it—you'll be able to figure out the interviewer's agenda, though it may never be clearly or overtly stated. Stop thinking about what you'll say next and pay close attention to what the other person is saying. As soon as their purpose becomes clear to you, you can start to tailor your responses to suit that purpose. Though they may never have said that they are looking for help in their project, for example, their detailing of the problems in their unit may prompt you to say: "Because of my experience as a nurse in a Children's Oncology unit I should be able to help in your new project."

Difficult Interviewers

It would be nice only to run into considerate, literate, kindly, interested, and interesting interviewers. Reality and experience tell us that this is not always the case. Here are three kinds of problem interviewers you might run across—and some suggestions on how to handle them.

All business. She's apt to be short-tempered and impatient, her desk piled high with work. She's too busy and has no appetite for pleasantries and no time for small talk. There's no use trying to win—or even begin—an argument with someone like this. Instead, refrain from being daunted by her abrupt manner, and instead pull out all the stops on your own store of patience and kindness. Sometimes this sort of interviewer tries to force your answers at an unreasonable speed. Her quick speech makes you feel you should reply in kind. Don't be tricked into this. Answer her questions at a thoughtful pace. If she throws three questions at you at once, pause and ask which she would like answered first. You can control the pace without seeming to be inconsiderate or uncooperative.

No business. This one doesn't talk, she barks out short questions and grunts in response. Every one of your answers is met with this type of noncommittal reply so you're left having to start from scratch each time. All you can do with such short questions and responses is have your answers be as full and detailed as you can make them. Don't let this type of interviewer put you off. These are often the most successful in terms of outcome.

If you choose to, you can even try to get the interviewer to elaborate by asking her a question that throws the ball back in her court; for example: "Is that the way you see it?"

Bad business. This interviewer is either new to the job or just not good at it. You wonder as you sit there how she was ever hired in the first place. She's not asking the right questions, and, if it keeps up this way, you're never going to be able to say what you want. The only thing to do is tactfully maneuver the conversation so you are in control. If you've prepared as carefully as you should have, you'll now have plenty to say. Just make sure to keep your mind on the goals you've set and be sensitive to the agenda the interviewer is trying, not very successfully, to put forth.

One way to turn the conversation in your direction is first to respond to her question, no matter how irrelevant it may be, and then go on and say what you have in mind. For example: "It's very interesting that you should mention cost, but, before we consider that, we have to look at the quality of the work. Now in my unit . . . "

Interview Tips

- Don't let the interviewer lead. When doing an interview, you do not have to be the victim of the person asking the questions. In fact, you may answer a question however you like. One way to do this is to pick out a key word in the interviewer's sentence and include it in your answer.
- Use the interviewer's name when you answer a question.
- Don't sit with your arms crossed over your chest. It makes you look defensive.
- Remember that keeping your hands folded in your lap makes you look meek.
- Take up space. Open up your body. Put your hands on the arm rests, lean back. Make your body asymmetrical: one hand on the arm of the chair, the other in your lap.
- When you've been asked a difficult question, resist the urge to fidget and shift positions.
- Don't stall for time by repeating the question.
- If there have been errors on your part, acknowledge them, then move beyond them. Don't try to back out of an obvious mistake. "Management dropped the ball on that one, but now that we understand how important it was to the staff, we mean to pay it serious attention in the future. As a matter of fact, our plan is to . . . "
- Take your time. Don't rush to answer until you know what you're going to say.
- Avoid using phrases like "uh" and "you know."
- Don't raise your voice at the end of your answer so that a statement sounds like a question.

- Keep your eyes on the interviewer and your hands away from your mouth.
- If you are part of a group interview, you should agree before-hand that everyone gets equal time, even if that requires prompt-ing of the shyest member.

THE TELEPHONE

Your job may be such that you spend a lot of time conducting business on the telephone. If this is so, you would do well to realize the inherent advantages so you can make the most of them, and the built-in disadvantages so you can minimize them.

Disadvantages

- You can't see the other person.
- You can't "read" their facial expressions or pick up clues as to their reaction from what they do with their body.
- You can't communicate with your face and body.
- You can't make creative use of silence. On the telephone, silence is always uncomfortable.

Advantages

- You can say what you want, get the other person's response, and get back to work, all without having left your desk.
- You have the potential to have better control over the way things are going, since you have only two elements to deal with: your voice and your attitude.
- You don't have to look your best.

Who's Calling?

The standard procedure for making a telephone call seems too obvious to repeat. When something is "too obvious to repeat" it usually means it's never repeated and, in fact, bears repeating.

- Identify yourself.
- Ask for the person with whom you wish to speak.
- State the reason for your call and how long it will take.
- Ask if the person you've called has time to speak with you now.
- Know the message you're going to leave, if the person is not there, or if a machine answers (your name, the time you called, the reason for your call, your intention—either to call back and at what time you'll do that, or to wait for their call, in which case leave your number and the best time to reach you).

Vocal Technique

- You have nothing to use but your voice. Make it work for you.
- Don't shout.
- Don't whisper.
- Speak with precision. People often rely on seeing another person's lips move to hear what they're saying. Without this to help them, you need to speak as clearly as you can.

Attitude

It carries in your voice. If you're angry, you'll sound angry. If you're smiling, that smile will communicate itself. If you're feeling stiff and uncomfortable, if you're reading from a prepared text rather than simply speaking as you would to someone sitting across the table, you'll sound that way, too.

- Imagine you can see the person you're talking to. Gesture in a natural way.
- Imagine they can see you. Just because they can't doesn't mean you can engage in unrelated physical activities while you're talking.
- Try staying on your feet as you talk, even walking around. It can help to keep your energy level high.
- Be sensitive to the circumstances of your call.

Do they want to hear from you?

Are they expecting your call, or dreading it?
Are you interrupting them?
Is your call coming just before lunch or just before the end of the work day?
Do you want something from them or are you offering them something?
Are you calling at home on a business matter? Or at the office on a personal matter?

Prepare To Make the Call

Don't waste time on time-saving calls. Huh? We all know what it's like to be involved in a piece of work and suddenly realize we need to know one piece of information and just who the person is who has it. Without another thought, we make the call and ask the question. Great. Except now that you have that information, you realize there's just one other thing you didn't know. But you can't call that same person back. You would have been better off letting the original question become part of a list and, later in the day, when the list was complete, making the call and asking all your questions.

Organize Your Ideas

Write everything down on a piece of paper before you call. If you're making the call to get information, write down all the questions you want to ask. It will be up to you to lead the conversation and the person you've called will be grateful for it.

Prepare Other Materials

This includes pen and paper for taking notes, charts, diagrams, definitions, order forms, references, telephone, and date book.
Think the conversation through before you make the call. Take into account every eventuality you can think of, and be ready for it.

Get to the Point

Although a certain amount of informal chit-chat may be appropriate when you're acquainted with the person you've called, you should not let this go on for too long. If the person you've called has to interrupt your inquiries about her state of health to say: "What can I do for you?" you have let the informal part of the conversation go on too long. In telephone communications, people appreciate someone who gets right to the point. (If you're the recipient of a call, however, you may speed things along by saying that very thing—"What can I do for you?"—especially if you know the person has a tendency to waste time in idle chatter.)

Dealing with Secretaries

Secretaries and administrative assistants are there to help you, but first they are there to help the person for whom they work. If they think they are helping their boss by making it difficult for you to get through, that is something you will have to deal with. The secretary may know that you are trying to get some information from her boss and that her boss has not yet put that information together. She may say her boss is not in, or is in a meeting, or is out of the office, or is unavailable to come to the phone. It will do you no good to take it personally, even though it may, in fact, be personal. If you've ever watched how many calls come to a secretary's desk, you will appreciate that keeping you waiting is an unavoidable part of the job.

Rather than take out your frustration on the secretary—who will not be on your side in this matter if you speak rudely to her—it is best to enlist her aid. Ask for her name in a friendly way, make a note of it, and use it whenever you speak to her. If you are having difficulty getting through to her boss, tell the secretary how difficult it's been for you and her boss to connect, tell her what you want from her boss, and ask the secretary's advice on how to accomplish it. Or, suggest a solution yourself and solicit her opinion. However you do it, make her your ally and she will become part of the solution, not part of the problem.

Listening

- Listening is not passive. Think of it as an activity.
- Encourage the speaker with occasional phrases such as "I see" or "of course."

- Repeat key words and phrases and write them down. Not only will this help you remember them later on, it will help you to focus your listening attention.
- If you have listened carefully, you have earned the right to interrupt. Be very specific when you do.

Answering

If a Martian were to look down on Earth, with no knowledge of Earth's customs, he would think it odd indeed that there was an instrument that sat near people no matter where they were and this instrument had such power that whenever it emitted a signal— *brrrrnnng! brrrrnnng!*—people stopped whatever they were doing, interrupted whomever they were talking to, put down whatever they were holding in their hands, and rushed to pick it up.

Such is the power of the telephone to command our attention—and so conditioned are we to obey—that the person who will not be interrupted by the telephone's ring—who will continue to do whatever it is they were doing when the telephone rang—is considered eccentric. How can you *not* answer the phone?

Nothing, it would seem, is so important that it cannot be interrupted to answer the telephone.

As long as that is the case—and as long as no one suggests an alternative—answering the telephone is an activity in which we all continue to be involved. And since we will, there are a few things we ought to know about how to answer the telephone.

When the telephone rings, we have no knowledge of who is calling. We may be expecting a particular person to call, but we don't really know until we pick up the telephone and the caller identifies herself.

Telephone-Answering Etiquette

Resist the impulse to answer as if you are certain who has called. "Hi Jean! I knew it was you!"—in which case you run the risk of the person (your boss? Con Ed? the salesman you were trying to avoid?) saying: "It's not Jean." Worse, you may have begun talking about something only that person would understand or should hear.

Instead, answer as if the person on the other end is the one you most want to impress with your best qualities. Your reasons for doing this may range from wanting to do business with that person, wanting that person to give you something, or do something for you, wanting to incur that person's good will for some unnamed and unknown favor that might be asked in the future, or wanting that person's cooperation for a cause or a venture that is more significant to you than to the caller.

If you are in the middle of a heated discussion with a lab technician, if you are frustrated with the pile-up of paperwork on your desk, if you are on a coffee break and laughing with a coworker, don't carry this tone over to answering the telephone.

When reaching for the telephone to answer a call, never assume that the caller is unimportant or indicate by your tone of voice that the person has interrupted you, or is bothering you. Remember one important fact: *you* answered the telephone. You did not have to answer the telephone. Don't answer it and then, by your tone—exasperation, impatience, unfriendly one-word replies—blame the person for interrupting you.

It is certainly within your rights to let this person know you are busy and have only a few minutes to spare. If she needs to talk for longer, ask if she can call you back at a time convenient to both of you. A logical person would rather talk to you when you can give her your complete attention. Depending on your relationship with the person, you may suggest calling her back, or ask if she can call you back. In either case, be specific about when the next call will take place.

Keep your mind on your goal, which is to effect the best communication possible between you and the other person, achieve and maintain an amicable relationship, and to get what you want.

The best way to avoid the kind of errors that come from 1) assuming you know who's calling, 2) demonstrating your annoyance at being interrupted, and 3) transferring your mood to the phone caller, is to have a standard manner in which you always answer the phone, one that sounds natural and relaxed. This will save you having to wonder if the way you are answering is appropriate to the caller. Your answer will be appropriate, no matter who that person is.

SPECIAL OCCASIONS

Presenting an Award

The occasion might be the honoring of a person's retirement, or a golden anniversary of service, or a particular mission successfully accomplished. The honoree may be your boss, colleague, rival, relative, or old friend. Whatever the occasion, and whatever your relationship to the person, be generous with your praise, be specific about their accomplishments, and personal about their personality and about your relationship. Relate an anecdote that only you, by virtue of your special relationship, would know, and how it demonstrates the very traits that are being awarded.

If you don't know the honoree personally, don't pretend you do; admit you only know her by reputation and what a fine reputation it is. If you have been inspired by her example, or learned from her work, say so.

Invocation

You may be called upon to speak at the dedication of a new building, or the inception of a new policy, or the induction of a new leader. Keep in mind that not all people in the audience may think or feel as you do in regard to this event; don't be so specific that you alienate anyone. Don't assume all believe as you do; instead, keep your words general and all embracing. Honor and pay respect to large issues with which no one may disagree: human dignity, a wish for world peace.

Commencement

When speaking at the graduation of the latest nursing class, remember that you're speaking to a group that is in a satisfied and joyous frame of mind. Also remember that it is a group—graduates, parents, and teachers alike—that is celebrating the completion of something. If they're wearing caps and gowns they're probably uncomfortable and so are the chairs they're sitting in. Don't keep them there any longer than you have to; they want to get out and celebrate. Your words should be inspirational and uplifting, a vision of their glorious future and the wonderful work upon which they are about to embark.

Introduction of a Speaker

If you've been called upon to introduce a speaker, the smartest first step is find out what he or she would like you to say. This applies, whether you know the person or not. Call them or write to them and get their input on the kinds of things they'd like you to say. They may be embarrassed to tell you, so you need to reassure them that this is not bragging on their part; they are simply furnishing you with the information you need to serve them best. The information you want is their full name—which you should mention several times in your introduction, the reason they are the one giving this particular speech, and the subject title of the speech. This is not a way to give the speaker's entire résumé, but to prepare the audience for who is going to be speaking to them.

Write this information in your own words. Keep it brief, to the point, and straightforward. You don't want to compete with the speaker by being too funny or too solemn, or by giving away the impact of their speech by touching on some of the points she'll be touching upon herself. You also don't want to oversell the speaker by telling the audience how fabulous she is or that she is the best, the wisest, and the funniest. A speaker who's been raised too high in audience expectations is set up to disappoint that audience.

Say the speaker's name at the beginning of your introduction, several times during your introduction, and at the very end. Then stay at the podium, dais, or wherever you are, until the speaker arrives. Shake her hand and go back to where you were sitting. (It pays to let the speaker know what the last line of your introduction is, so she'll be ready to stand.)

There are several ways *not* to introduce a speaker, phrases that have become so overused they have lost all meaning:

"We have a speaker here today who needs no introduction."

"We are truly honored to have with us today."

"And so, without further ado . . . "
"On this most memorable occasion."

Impromptu Speaking

Even before you go to the event, you have a general idea of the topics that will be spoken about. You'll probably know who the speakers are and, if you don't, you'll know as soon as you arrive, when you'll also learn the topic of their speeches. By the time the speech begins—and certainly by the time it's over—you'll know a lot about the audience, as well. If you're an interested listener, you'll probably have responses as the speakers are talking. Speaking impromptu is nothing more than stating that response.

You may be asked to speak from the floor. You may have a question to ask the speaker. You may be singled out as a representative of your group, or because of your own expertise in the field being spoken about or a related field.

The first thing to remember is: don't feel you have to speak. If the prospect of speaking without being prepared terrifies you . . . if you weren't listening . . . if you missed part of the speech . . . if you have no strong feeling one way or the other . . . if, for whatever reason, you simply have nothing to say, or don't feel that what you do have to say will be illuminating, informative, or noteworthy or will reflect well on you . . . there is nothing wrong with simply saying that you need some time to think about your response and, once having taken that time, will perhaps speak later.

If you do have something to say, make sure you start with a clear idea. Jot down a few key words to which you may refer. In your eagerness to be heard, don't take the floor and then search for what you want to say.

Using Media Technology

Technology is providing more sophisticated ways of communicating with an audience: videoconferencing, satellite distribution, laser discs and pointers, CD ROM transmission, and videotaped programs. All of this means that making a simple presentation is no longer as simple as it used to be. You may be talking in front of an audience of nurse managers in a hotel ballroom in Chicago at the same time you're being seen via satellite in hospitals and class-rooms all across the country. In today's high-tech world, resistance to these kind of techniques can only limit a speaker's effectiveness. Embracing these tools can enhance it.

It is no longer enough to show a slide and hold a pointer to it. Today's audiences are technologically sophisticated. They're prepared to see new technologies like video projections and com-puter-generated graphics. Using these as part of your repertoire of special effects can make your presentation deliver what it promises. Think of technology as one more piece of equipment that is going to help you communicate your ideas. Don't use a technique just because it's the latest gadget on the communications market. And don't be intimidated by those who do. Ultimately it is the content of your speech that makes the impact. Use technology, don't let technology use you.

Speaking on Television

Not every televised speaker appears on the *David Letterman Show*. There are many situations in which you may be asked to speak in front of a television camera: as part of a news story, as part of a documentary about your specialty, the videotaped recording of a speech you're making live, the videotaping of a lecture you've given a hundred times before. In other words, you may be invited to speak with plenty of time to prepare; you may be speaking already and only have to make adjustments for the camera; you may be interrupted in your work to speak extemporaneously.

If it is a regularly scheduled show, watch the show before you appear on it. Learn about the host and the format and the way guests are treated. Arrive on the set early enough to get the lay of the land. Sit where you'll be sitting during the broadcast or taping, and make sure you're comfortable and not sinking into the upholstery. Check and see that your eyes aren't badly affected by the television lights and that your glasses don't reflect light at the camera. (Ask the cameraman.) Be prepared to do the show without your glasses.

When you're on the set, ask what the camera will be focused on. If it is a close-up of your face, there is no point making clarifying gestures with your hands or holding up an object to explain yourself if that portion of your anatomy will not be seen. Find out how long you have to speak, if there are other guests as well as you, if people are going to call in and ask questions, if the host or hostess of the show is knowledgeable about the topic, or even if they are hostile or confrontative about it, and if you're going to be provided with the questions the moderator might ask.

Don't wear white. Video lights are "hot." White will actually create a buzz when the image is transmitted. Wear neutral solid colors; television transmission itself is composed of horizontal bands, which tend to flatten the image and, because the lights are hot, subtle colors and patterns tend not to register as well as primary colors and shapes.

When the show is on, maintain your focus. There will be activity behind the camera that might attract your attention. Don't let it. Don't look the camera in the eye. Keep your head up. Television picks up every gesture, every subtle nuance that an audience in a banquet hall doesn't. Play to this close-up scrutiny; keep gestures intimate. Speak clearly and conversationally. Try as much as you can to couch your answers as coming from your own experience, either personal or professional.

If you don't like the question—if it is too general, if it boxes you into a formulaic answer, if it's a trap—answer one you do like, even if it hasn't been asked. See unwanted questions as an opportunity. You have the floor and, with a few subtle changes, you can turn a hostile or trick question into an interesting and positive answer.

CONCLUSION

Most of what you've read in this book is a matter of common sense because, if you've ever had a conversation with another human being, you've already spoken in public. To be an effective, compelling, dynamic speaker is not a gift that other people have; it is nothing more—or less—than a series of skills that can be read about, studied, learned, and applied.

As you've seen throughout these pages, most of what there is to be learned about speaking in public is already within your experience as a nurse. What this book has done is codify that experience for you, demonstrated how to marshal the public-speaking skills you already have, how to identify those skills you need to develop, and how to bring them together to realize your full potential in oral communication.

Appendix:
Speech Checklist

WHAT TO KNOW BEFORE YOU GO

- Know where you're going to be.
- Know the occasion.
- Know who you're talking to.
- Know how long you have.

PREPARE YOUR SPEECH

- Compose one concise sentence that clearly states your purpose.
- Construct an outline.
- Write the speech.
- Plan your visuals.

PREPARE YOURSELF

- Practice the speech.
- Decide how to look.
- Make a checklist of what to bring.
- Get directions.
- Get there early.

BEFORE THE MEETING

- Communicate with meeting planners.
- Check the physical layout.

- Check the technical equipment.
- Find out where you're supposed to be right before you speak.
- Find out what you do right after you speak.

MAKE THE SPEECH

- Look the audience square in the eye.
- Start talking.
   Tell them what you're going to tell them.
   Then tell them.
   Then tell them what you just told them.
- Use the microphone.
   Don't bend to meet it, or let it block your face, or speak
   while turned away from it.
- Use your visual aids.
   Illustrate only what is essential and hard to visualize.
   Talk to your audience, not your display.
   Avoid small details.
- Use the pointer sparingly. Put it down when you're not using it.
- Use natural gestures.
   Talk to the audience like you would talk to a friend.
- Use your voice like a tool.
   Vary your pitch, rate, and volume, and don't talk too fast.
- Ask for questions.
- When you're done, accept the applause with a smile, spot your
   exit, and go directly to it.

Bibliography

Booher, D. (1994). *Communicate with Confidence*. New York: McGraw-Hill.

Byrne, R. (1988). *1911 Best Things Anybody Ever Said*. New York: Fawcett.

Carnegie, D. (1956). *How to Develop Self-Confidence and Influence People by Public Speaking*. New York: Pocket Books.

Detz, J. (1992). *How to Write and Give a Speech*. New York: St. Martin's/Griffin.

Huff, R. (1992). *I Can See You Naked*. Kansas City, MO: Andrews & McNeel.

Lyle, G. R., & Guinagh, K. (1968). *I Am Happy to Present*. New York: H. W. Wilson.

Roan, C. (1995). *Speak Easy*. Washington, DC: Starrhill Press.

Schloff, L., & Yudkin, M. (1993). *Smart Speaking*. New York: Plume.

Walters, L. (1993). *Secrets of Successful Speakers*. New York: McGraw-Hill.

Wilder, L. (1986). *Professionally Speaking*. New York: Simon & Schuster.

Index

103

📮 *Springer Publishing Company*

Writing and Getting Published
A Primer for Nurses
Barbara Stevens Barnum, RN, PhD, FAAN

This book, by one of nursing's most accomplished authors, is a step-by-step guide to developing professional writing skills and navigating the publication process. It includes pointers on structuring one's writing, avoiding common mistakes, making a term paper or dissertation publishable, writing query letters and book proposals, and finding and working with a publisher. The ability to communicate effectively in writing is an important tool for sharing knowledge and expertise, and for advancing a career. This concise guide demystifies the skills and procedures necessary to make this happen.

Contents:

Part I. Writing the Article • Finding the Right Topic • Writing the Article • Avoiding Common Mistakes • It's a Great Term Paper: Why Don't You Get it Published? • Publication Options: Sending Your Article to the Right Journal • What about a Query Letter? • Submitting Articles: Getting the Procedures Right • When Your Article Reaches the Journal

Part II. Writing the Book • How Book Writing Differs from Article Writing • The Edited or Coauthored Book • It's a Great Dissertation, But is it a Book? • Producing the Book Prospectus • Finding and Working with a Publisher

Part III. Special Issues • Writing with Colleagues • Writing from Research • Writing about Work Instruments

Appendices • Appendix A: List of Nursing Journals • Appendix B: List of Nursing Book Publishers • Appendix C: Additional Writing Resources

1995   216pp   0-8261-8690-4   hardcover

536 Broadway, New York, NY 10012-3955 • (212) 431-4370 • Fax (212) 941-7842

SP *Springer Publishing Company*

SUCCESSFUL GRANT WRITING
Strategies for Health and Human Service Professionals

Laura N. Gitlin, PhD and **Kevin J. Lyons,** PhD

This book guides the reader through the language and basic components of grantmanship. It illustrates how to develop ideas for funding, write the sections of a proposal, organize different types of project structures, and finally, how to understand the review process.

Each chapter describes a specific aspect of grantmanship and suggests innovative strategies to implement the information that

> SUCCESSFUL
> GRANT
> WRITING
>
> *Strategies for Health and*
> *Human Service Professionals*
>
> LAURA N. GITLIN, PHD
> KEVIN J. LYONS, PHD
>
> **SP**
> *Springer Publishing Company*

is presented. The appendices contain helpful materials, such as a list of key acronyms, examples of timelines and sample budget sheets. The strategies in this volume are beneficial to individuals and departments in academic, clinical, or community-based settings.

Partial Contents:
- Becoming Familiar with Funding Sources
- Developing Your Ideas for Funding
- Learning about Your Institution
- Common Sections of Proposals
- Preparing a Budget
- Technical Considerations
- Strategies for Effective Writing
- Understanding the Process of Collaboration
- Understanding the Review Process

1996   235pp   0-8261-9260-2   hard cover

536 Broadway, New York, NY 10012-3955 • (212) 431-4370 • Fax (212) 941-7842

$\mathcal{SP}$ *Springer Publishing Company*

TEACHING CREATIVELY WITH VIDEO
Fostering Reflection, Communication and other Clinical Skills

Jane Westberg, PhD, and
Hilliard Jason, MD, EdD, Editors

"This book is a 'must-read' for the serious medical teacher who wants to achieve a full measure of professionalism via mastery of all the tools of the art. Westberg and Jason are master teachers who have pioneered the use of video over more than three decades.

The book concisely describes a philosophy of collaborative trust-based education within which video can be a most powerful tool."
                                                    —**Michael K. Magill**, MD,
                    Tallahassee Memorial Regional Medical Center

Contents:

Introduction: Managing Instructional Challenges

I: Using Video in the Classroom. Using Video for Illustrating, Modeling, and Demonstrating • Selecting and Using Video Triggers • Making and Reviewing Tapes of Role-Played Exercises

II: Using Video in Clinical Supervision. Preparing for and Making Recordings • Helping Learners Use Video for Reflection and Self-Assessment • Using Video for Providing Constructive Feedback • Helping Learners Use Video for Peer Review • Eliciting Patients' Perspectives

Springer Series on Medical Education
1994   256pp   0-8261-8360-3   hardcover

536 Broadway, New York, NY 10012-3955 • (212) 431-4370 • Fax (212) 941-7842

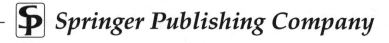

Springer Publishing Company

The Nurse Consultant's Handbook

Belinda Puetz, PhD, RN
Linda J. Shinn, MBA, RN, CAE

What is a consultant? What type of person makes a successful consultant? How does one launch and manage one's own business as a consultant? This manual answers these questions and provides comprehensive guidelines and practical information on becoming a nurse consultant.

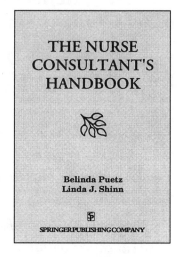

The authors, both experienced consultants, outline the consultation process in detail, describe the business and financial savvy required, and give tips on marketing and pricing one's services, making presentations, networking, and managing one's personal life in relation to one's career. The book addresses independent entrepreneurs as well as "intrapreneurs" who consult as an inside member of a larger organization.

Contents:
- What is Consultation?
- The Consultation Process
- Preparation for Consultation: Planning a Career Path
- The Internal Nurse Consultant
- Starting a Consulting Business
- Marketing Consultation Services
- Networking
- Legal and Ethical Aspects of Consulting
- The Consultant as a Person

1997   248pp   0-8261-9520-2   Hard

536 Broadway, New York, NY 10012-3955 • (212) 431-4370 • Fax (212) 941-7842